Pocket Guide to Stress Testing

Pocket Guide to Stress Testing

Second Edition

Edited by

Dennis A. Tighe, MD, FACP, FACC, FASE
Associate Director, Noninvasive Cardiology
Director, Adult Congenital Heart Disease Clinic
Professor of Medicine
Division of Cardiovascular Medicine
University of Massachusetts Medical School
Worcester, MA, USA

Bryon A. Gentile, II, MD, FACC
Assistant Professor of Medicine
Division of Cardiovascular Medicine
University of Massachusetts Medical School
Worcester, MA, USA

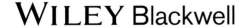

This edition first published 2020 © 2020 by John Wiley & Sons Ltd.
Edition History [1e, 1997]

Registered Office(s)
John Wiley & Sons, Inc., 111 River Street, Hoboken, NJ 07030, USA
John Wiley & Sons Ltd, The Atrium, Southern Gate, Chichester, West Sussex, PO19 8SQ, UK

Editorial Office
9600 Garsington Road, Oxford, OX4 2DQ, UK

For details of our global editorial offices, customer services, and more information about Wiley products visit us at www.wiley.com.

Wiley also publishes its books in a variety of electronic formats and by print-on-demand. Some content that appears in standard print versions of this book may not be available in other formats.

Limit of Liability/Disclaimer of Warranty

Library of Congress Cataloging-in-Publication Data
Names: Tighe, Dennis A., editor. | Gentile, Bryon A., II, editor. | Preceded by (work): Chung, Edward K. Pocket guide to stress testing.
Title: Pocket guide to stress testing / edited by Dennis A. Tighe, Bryon A. Gentile, II.
Description: Second edition. | Hoboken, NJ: Wiley, 2020. | Preceded by Pocket guide to stress testing / Edward K. Chung, Dennis A. Tighe. c1997. |
    Includes bibliographical references and index.
Identifiers: LCCN 2019024458 | ISBN 9781119481775 (paperback) | ISBN 9781119481799 (adobe pdf) | ISBN 9781119481751 (epub)
Subjects: | MESH: Exercise Test | Electrocardiography | Heart Diseases–diagnosis | Handbook
Classification: LCC RC683.5.S77 | NLM WG 39 | DDC 616.1/207543–dc23
LC record available at https://lccn.loc.gov/2019024458

Cover Design: Wiley
Cover Image: © Bryon Gentile

Set in 10/12pt Warnock by SPi Global, Pondicherry, India
Printed and bound in Singapore by Markono Print Media Pte Ltd

10 9 8 7 6 5 4 3 2 1

To my wife, Leslie, and our children, Elizabeth and Alexander
—Dennis A. Tighe

To my wife, Kaitlin, and our children, Cecelia and Caroline
—Bryon A. Gentile

Contents

Contributors

Seth T. Dahlberg, MD, FACC
Associate Professor of Medicine
Division of Cardiovascular Medicine
University of Massachusetts Medical School
Worcester, MA, USA

John B. Dickey, MD
Assistant Professor of Medicine
Division of Cardiovascular Medicine
University of Massachusetts Medical School
Worcester, MA, USA

Bryon A. Gentile, II, MD, FACC
Assistant Professor of Medicine
Division of Cardiovascular Medicine
University of Massachusetts Medical School
Worcester, MA, USA

Samuel A.E. Headley, PhD, FACSM
Professor, Exercise Science and Sport Studies
Springfield College
Springfield, MA, USA

Thomas W. Rowland, MD, FAAP, FACSM
Retd. Director, Pediatric Cardiology
Baystate Medical Center
Springfield, MA, USA
Associate Professor of Pediatrics
Tufts University School of Medicine
Boston, MA, USA

Dennis A. Tighe, MD, FACP, FACC, FASE
Associate Director, Noninvasive Cardiology
Director, Adult Congenital Heart Disease Clinic
Professor of Medicine
Division of Cardiovascular Medicine
University of Massachusetts Medical School
Worcester, MA, USA

Preface

Since the first edition of the *Pocket Guide* was published, the role of stress testing in evaluating patients with suspected cardiovascular disease has been affirmed and new indications have emerged. In addition, new information on the application of stress testing in specific patient populations and the role of myocardial imaging in conjunction with stress testing has continued to evolve. Thus, the impetus for this second edition was to update the reader on the proper application, performance, and interpretation of the various stress testing modalities used in the contemporary stress laboratory. Each chapter has been revised to reflect the most up-to-date information available.

Although abundant information and expansive texts on stress testing are available, we believe that the success of the first edition of the *Pocket Guide* stemmed from its focused content, emphasis on key points, and inclusion of informative illustrations and tables. Therefore, in the second edition we intentionally continued using a format that is bulleted and focused, and makes extensive use of tables and illustrations to present the essential information without over-emphasizing esoteric points. We also include a list of key references in the field at the end of each chapter, so that the reader requiring more detailed information can explore topics of interest in greater depth.

As indications and applications for stress testing have evolved, so has the number of non-physician healthcare professionals involved in the assessment of patients prior to stress testing, during actual performance and monitoring of the test, and issuing of preliminary interpretation of test results. Given the subject matter and practical information included, this edition of the *Pocket Guide* should prove to be a valuable resource to both physicians and non-physicians involved in the care of these patients.

I would like to acknowledge the contributions of my colleagues, who have provided insightful and up-to-date information. My co-author, Bryon A. Gentile, II, deserves special recognition for his contribution of many valuable and highly informative chapters; without his efforts this edition of the *Pocket Guide* would not have been possible. I wish to acknowledge the staff of Wiley Publishers for their support and cooperation during the process of bringing this project to fruition.

Finally, I wish to pay special recognition posthumously to my mentor, teacher, co-author, and friend, Edward K. Chung, MD. Dr. Chung was an internationally recognized author and leader in the field of electrocardiography and all its applications. He was a generous teacher who demanded excellence and influenced a generation of learners in the heart station at the Thomas Jefferson University Hospital. I was particularly fortunate to have known him and learned from him. It was my distinct privilege to have co-authored the first edition of the *Pocket Guide* with him. I will be forever grateful to him for his wisdom and encouragement.

Dennis A. Tighe, MD
Worcester, MA, USA

Abbreviations

ACC	American College of Cardiology		EF	Ejection fraction
ACLS	Advance cardiac life support		FDA	Food and Drug Administration
ACSM	American College of Sports Medicine		HF	Heart failure
AHA	American Heart Association		HFpEF	Heart failure with preserved ejection fraction
APC	Atrial premature contraction		HFrEF	Heart failure with reduced ejection fraction
ASCVD	Atherosclerotic cardiovascular disease		HLA	Horizontal long-axis
AT	Atrial tachycardia		HR	Heart rate
AV	Atrioventricular		HRR	Heart rate reserve
BLS	Basic life support		Hz	Hertz
BP	Blood pressure		IV	intravenous
bpm	beats per minute		kg	kilogram
BSA	Body surface area		LBBB	Left bundle branch block
CAD	Coronary artery disease		LV	Left ventricle
CHF	Congestive heart failure		LVH	Left ventricular hypertrophy
CPX	Cardiopulmonary exercise test		MAC	Maximal aerobic capacity
DBP	Diastolic blood pressure		METs	Metabolic equivalents
DTS	Duke treadmill score		mg	milligram
ECC	Emergency cardiovascular care		MI	Myocardial infarction
ECG	Electrocardiogram		ml	milliliter

mph	miles per hour	rpm	revolutions per minute
MPI	Myocardial perfusion imaging	RVG	Radionuclide ventriculography
NPO	nothing per oral	SA	Short-axis
MVPS	Mitral valve prolapse syndrome	SBP	Systolic blood pressure
NYHA	New York Heart Association	SPECT	Single photon emission computed
PACS	Picture archiving and communication system		tomographic
PAG	Physical activity guidelines for Americans	SV	Stroke volume
PET	Positron emission tomographic	VLA	Vertical long-axis
Q	Cardiac output	VO_{2max}	maximal/peak oxygen uptake
RBBB	Right bundle branch block	VPC	Ventricular premature contraction
RER	Respiratory exchange ratio	VT	Ventricular tachycardia
RPE	Rate of perceived exertion	WPW	Wolff-Parkinson-White

1 Introduction

Dennis A. Tighe

Introduction

The stress (exercise) ECG test serves as an important and valuable assessment tool that provides diagnostic and prognostic information in the clinical evaluation and management of patients with known or suspected cardiovascular disease, particularly coronary artery disease (CAD).

Various protocols for exercise stress testing have been in in existence for several decades. Early protocols for exercise testing, such as Master's two-step test, lacked sufficient sensitivity for clinical use. Currently in the United States, exercise electrocardiography is most commonly performed using a motor-driven treadmill. In Europe, where bicycling is more habitual, exercise stress testing is more commonly performed using a bicycle ergometer.

Several multistage exercise ECG testing protocols have been developed for use with either a motorized treadmill (the Bruce protocol or its modification are the most widely used in the United States) or cycle ergometer (see Chapter 5).

For those unable to perform sufficient physical exertion to adequately complete an exercise ECG test, or when specific clinical conditions exist, pharmacological stress testing with vasodilators or dobutamine is indicated (see Chapter 8). Among patients with resting ECG abnormalities expected to affect repolarization that potentially lead to situations where the ECG response to exercise would be considered non-diagnostic or falsely positive, imaging with echocardiography or myocardial perfusion imaging (MPI) is indicated. Stress echocardiography is also indicated in specific situations in the assessment of valvular heart disease (see Chapter 7). For selected patients with indwelling permanent cardiac pacemakers, the gradual increase of the atrial paced rate can provide an adequate assessment for myocardial ischemia when combined with a myocardial imaging technique.

The exercise ECG test is used primarily to assess the etiology of chest pain and for detection of CAD. In addition, the exercise ECG test can provide important information about functional capacity (prognosis) and the efficacy of medical and surgical therapy for patients with CAD. Furthermore, an exercise ECG test can be quite useful in assessing the ability of an individual to participate in an exercise program or sport (see Chapters 18 and 19), in the evaluation exercise-related symptoms, or for assessment of chronotropic competence or exercise-related arrhythmias.

Myocardial imaging should be performed in combination with the exercise ECG test when false positive or false negative exercise ECG results are anticipated or found and when the exercise ECG test result is equivocal. Due to the infrequent occurrence of ST-segments shifts with pharmacological stress agents, myocardial imaging is required when pharmacological stress testing is performed (see Chapter 11).

Pathophysiologic Considerations

The exercise stress ECG test has two major purposes:

1) To determine the capability of the coronary circulation to increase oxygen delivery to the myocardium in response to an increased demand. During physical exertion, myocardial oxygen demand is increased by the increase in systolic blood pressure (SBP), contractile state of the heart, and increase of heart rate (HR).
2) To assess the exercise capacity. The major factor determining the exercise capacity is the ability to increase the cardiac output; the product of stroke volume (SV) and HR. In normal individuals, cardiac output (Q) typically increases by a factor of four to sixfold from the resting condition to peak exercise. During moderate to high-intensity exercise, the further increase in Q is primarily attributable to an increase in HR, as SV generally reaches a plateau at 50–60% of maximal oxygen uptake.

As it is known that the heart already extracts approximately 70% of the oxygen from each unit of blood perfusing the myocardium at rest, oxygen delivery to the myocardium cannot be increased significantly by increasing oxygen extraction. For practical purposes, myocardial metabolism is entirely aerobic, thus coronary blood flow must increase in order to augment the myocardial oxygen supply. In healthy individuals, coronary blood flow is documented to increase in proportion to increased myocardial demand for oxygen.

In response to stress in patients with significant CAD, coronary blood flow fails to adequately increase to meet the increased demand of the myocardium for oxygen, leading to myocardial ischemia. Myocardial ischemia may manifest in a variety of ways during a stress test including anginal pain, ST-segment and/or T-wave changes, ventricular dysfunction, various cardiac arrhythmias, or any combination of the preceding.

Physical exercise leads to an increment of myocardial oxygen consumption via the increased HR, intra-myocardial tension, and contractility. With progressive exercise, coronary blood flow can increase as much as four to sixfold above the basal value. Acceleration of the HR is associated with a linear increment of myocardial oxygen consumption; thus the HR response to an exercise bout provides a useful parameter of myocardial oxygen requirements. By measuring the (systolic) BP during exercise, the product of the HR and BP ("double product" or "rate-pressure product") can be derived, which can serve as a practical index of myocardial oxygen uptake.

Preparations and Precautions

As shall be discussed in further detail in Chapter 2, the exercise ECG test requires certain preparations and due consideration of precautions in order to perform the test appropriately and safely. The nature and purpose of the test should be explained in appropriate detail to the patient. All stress tests must be ordered by a licensed independent practitioner. Upon receipt and acceptance of the order by the stress laboratory, the stress test is scheduled as an elective procedure for outpatients as well as for inpatients.

Patients who are to undergo a stress test should be given the following instructions:

- Report for the test either after an overnight fast or three hours following a light meal.
- Routine medications may be taken with small amounts of water.
- Dress in comfortable clothing and wear comfortable walking shoes or sneakers.

Before a patient is to perform a stress test, the following procedures must be performed:

- A witnessed informed consent document must be obtained by the professional performing/supervising the stress test. This is an important medico-legal requirement (see Chapter 21). Translation services should be provided for non–English-speaking patients.

- A brief history and physical examination should be performed to determine whether the patient is suitable for the proposed test.
- The indication(s) for the test along with any potential contraindication(s) which may exist (see Chapters 3 and 4) should be carefully considered
- Determine whether the patient is taking any medication (e.g. beta-blockers, organic nitrates, calcium channel blockers, digitalis preparation, etc.) that may influence the result(s) of the stress test (see Chapter 15).

The following precautions should be observed prior to initiation of the stress test:

- Maintain the exercise stress laboratory at a comfortable temperature, generally between 68° and 72 °F, with 40–60% humidity.
- Instruct the patient in full regarding the stress test procedure.
- Have the patient rest comfortably in the supine position for a period of 5–10 minutes before the test is performed.
- A standard 12-lead ECG (supine and standing) should be obtained to determine the presence of any acute cardiac events (ECG changes) or any possible contraindications. The modified lead placement with the Mason-Likar ("torso") system used during stress may alter the inferior lead complexes to either mimic or hide previous Q waves.
- The stress test should be supervised by a licensed, qualified healthcare professional fully familiar with all aspects of the procedure, including use of the equipment, test interpretation, and recognition of potential complications that may arise. If a non-physician (nurse, nurse practitioner, physician assistant, exercise physiologist) is designated to supervise the stress test, a physician skilled in stress testing should be immediately available in the vicinity for consultation and assistance should such a situation arise.

During the test, the procedure should be halted immediately if either of the following occurs:

- The patient requests that the test stop.
- The patient develops significant symptoms (e.g. chest pain, dizziness, dyspnea, etc.), hypotension, cyanosis, bradycardia, or other serious cardiac arrhythmias and/or marked ST-segment changes.

Anyone supervising a stress test must be prepared for emergency situations:

- Although a rare occurrence, all necessary equipment for cardiac resuscitation must be immediately available in the stress laboratory.
- Treating patients immediately for significant symptoms, cardiac arrhythmias, and any other untoward complications.

The staff supervising the stress test must inspect all emergency equipment on a daily basis to ensure that any serious complication can be managed immediately, and all qualified healthcare personnel working in the stress laboratory must be capable of handling any cardiopulmonary emergencies (see Chapter 13).

Methodology

Methods of Stress

- *Exercise (stress) ECG test*. A motor-driven treadmill is the most commonly used device in the United States. Can also be accomplished using a cycle ergometer (more popular in Europe) or an arm ergometer (not commonly utilized).
- *Pharmacological stress testing*. Vasodilators (dipyridamole, adenosine, and regadenoson) or a catecholamine (dobutamine) can be used for those unable to perform an exercise stress test or in specific clinical situations (see Chapters 8 and 11).
- *Artificial pacing*. In selected patients with an indwelling cardiac pacemaker, the device can be used increase HR and assess for inducible myocardial ischemia. In rare instances today, a swallowed pill electrode can be used to pace the heart.

Protocols for the Treadmill Exercise ECG Test

As will be discussed further in Chapter 5, a number of multistage exercise protocols have been devised. In clinical practice, the Bruce protocol is employed most widely. Among certain subsets of patients or for specific clinical situations, an exercise protocol other than the Bruce protocol may be the more appropriate choice.

Planning the Ideal Exercise ECG Stress Test

- The initial workload should be within an individual's anticipated physical working capacity. Workloads should be increased gradually, not abruptly, and should be maintained for a sufficient length of time (generally three minutes) to attain a near physiological study state.
- Continuously monitoring HR, ST-segments, and cardiac rhythm during exercise is essential as is measuring BP during each stage. In addition, it is important to monitor the patient for signs and symptoms (chest pain, dyspnea, dizziness, extreme fatigue, perceived exertion) which may develop during an exercise bout as these may presage development of significant ECG changes or hemodynamic issues. As some abnormal responses occur after exercise, monitoring should continue for six to eight minutes in the post-exercise recovery period, or longer, if the patient is symptomatic or if BP, HR, and/or ST-segments have not returned to near-baseline values.
- An exercise ECG test is most often designed to be "symptom-limited;" most tests should be terminated because of fatigue, significant symptoms, and/or ECG changes rather than attainment of a particular HR goal.
- The exercise ECG test should be terminated immediately if significantly abnormal symptoms, marked ST-segment changes, serious arrhythmias, or significant shifts in blood pressure are found.

Choosing the Exercise ECG Protocol

As stated above, a variety of multistage protocols exist; the Bruce protocol is most widely used.

- With some exercise ECG protocols, workload is increased by changing speed alone while maintaining a fixed grade (incline or elevation).
- In the Bruce protocol, the workload is changed incrementally by increasing both the speed and grade of the treadmill.
- For the progressive increment of workload, three-minute intervals are preferable so that steady-state BP and HR responses can be achieved.
- A submaximal ("low-level") exercise ECG test protocol is recommended by some cardiologists in the setting of a stable patient following a recent myocardial infarction (MI) or acute coronary syndrome without full revascularization.

Metabolic equivalents (METs), multiples of the basal metabolic rate (1 MET is defined as ≈ 3.5 mlO$_2$ per kilogram of body weight per minute [ml/kg/min]), are commonly used to express the workload in various stages of the exercise ECG testing protocols.

- In the majority of patients with CAD, a workload of 8 METs is often sufficient for evaluation of angina pectoris.
- Healthy sedentary subjects are seldom able to exercise beyond a workload of 10–11 METs.
- Physically active individuals may be capable of achieving workloads in excess of 16 METs.

When correlating cardiac functional capacity with exercise workload expressed in METs, the following relationships are generally observed:

- Functional class III patients often become symptomatic at a workload of 3–4 METs.
- Functional class II patients often are limited by symptoms at workloads of 5–6 METs.
- Functional class I patients should be capable of achieving workloads in excess of 7–8 METs.

Lead System and Electrode Placement

Electrodes

Obtaining high-quality ECG recordings is the most important aspect for proper interpretation of the ECG stress test. Using appropriate electrodes and proper skin preparation at the site of electrode placement are essential.

- A disposable silver-silver chloride electrode that provides a good skin contact by means of a liquid conductor is the most reliable and optimal electrode.
- Proper skin preparation designed to remove the superficial oils and layer of skin to significantly lower resistance consists of:
  - Cleaning the sites of electrode application with ethyl alcohol.
  - Removing the superficial keratinized layer of epidermis by gentle abrasion.
  - Washing away the removed superficial epidermal layer by a light cleaning such as with acetone.

For the interface between the skin and electrode to be optimal, skin resistance should be reduced to $5000\,\Omega$ or less. After electrode placement, the technician should tap lightly on the electrode to assess adequacy of skin preparation (no noise on the ECG should be created with the tap).

In addition, efforts should be taken to minimize motion at the electrode-cable interface. This may be achieved by creating stress loops with precut tape strips or securing the cables centrally with an elastic belt worn around the waist. Disposable mesh vests placed on the upper torso can help secure the electrodes.

For women, particularly those with large breasts, a breast support garment should be worn during the exercise ECG test in order to minimize motion artifacts which can obscure diagnostic ECG changes and hide potentially dangerous arrhythmias during exercise.

Lead Systems

While historically single-channel lead systems such as monitoring lead V5 or bipolar lead CM5 were demonstrated to have high sensitivity for detecting myocardial ischemia compared to 12-lead ECG recordings, current systems utilize multiple ECG leads.

- Use of multiple leads has been shown to increase test sensitivity.
- In recording systems using multiple leads, the lateral precordial leads (leads V4 through V6) are capable of detecting 90% of all instances of ST-segment depression.
- In our laboratory, we monitor leads II, V1, and V5 continuously during stress and recovery. At the end of each stage (and periodically as required), a 12-lead ECG can be displayed and printed.
- The Mason-Likar ("torso") modification of lead placement is used during exercise to minimize muscle and motion artifact.

Observation

Most laboratories continue to use visual observation and interpretation (see Chapter 14) of the exercise ECG. Most modern ECG systems used for exercise testing collect data that would allow for computerized assessment of the exercise ECG test, particularly ST-segment abnormalities, which may enhance the predictive accuracy of the test (see Chapter 20).

Endpoints to Terminate Exercise ECG Stress Tests

A detailed description of the endpoints for the exercise ECG test is provided in Chapter 5. In general, a symptom-limited test (rather than a HR-limited test) to near-maximum level gives the most diagnostic information as well as providing assessment of exercise capacity/prognosis.

The qualified healthcare professional supervising the test must be able to make a correct, instant decision for each patient as to whether the exercise bout should continue or be terminated.

- Encourage the patient to continue when it is apparent that a lack of motivation is present and all parameters show expected (normal) findings.
- It is important to speak with the patient intermittently and to observe facial expression during exercise. These actions may help to assess whether the patient may have any unusual distress. Patients may try to overcome serious symptoms and not report them to the test supervisor.

When to Terminate the Exercise Prematurely

Patient-determined and provider-determined indications are recognized. Absolute indications include:

- The patient requests that the test stop.
- Significant symptoms, such as chest pain, dizziness, marked dyspnea, or severe fatigue, are produced.
- Signs such as ataxia, pallor, or cyanosis are observed.
- The patient experiences symptoms of an intensity that would prompt stopping daily activities. Do not insist that the patient continue on to reach a predicted HR.
- The patient develops ST-segment elevation (>1.0 mm) in leads without pre-existing Q waves because of prior MI (exceptions: leads aVR, aVL, and V1).
- Occurrence of severe cardiac arrhythmias, such as sustained ventricular tachycardia (VT) or other arrhythmia, including second- or third-degree atrioventricular block, preventing normal maintenance of cardiac output during exercise.
- A decline in systolic BP >10 mmHg occurs despite an increase in workload, when accompanied by any other evidence of myocardial ischemia.
- Development of technical difficulties in the monitoring/interpreting of the ECG or BP.

Relative indications include:

- Marked ST-segment displacement (horizontal or downsloping of >2 mm, measured 60–80 ms after the J point) in a patient with suspected ischemia.
- A decline in systolic BP >10 mmHg (persistently below baseline) despite an increase in workload, in the absence of other evidence of myocardial ischemia.
- Presence of arrhythmias other than sustained VT, including multifocal ventricular ectopy, ventricular triplets, supraventricular tachycardia, and bradyarrhythmias with the potential to become more complex or cause hemodynamic instability.
- Occurrence of an exaggerated hypertensive response, defined as SBP >250 mmHg or diastolic BP >115 mmHg.
- Development of bundle branch block that cannot immediately be distinguished from VT.

Indications Versus Contraindications (see Chapters 3 and 4)

Major Indications of the Exercise ECG Test

- Confirmation or exclusion of CAD; assessment of the etiology of chest pain or equivalent symptom.
- Assessment of functional capacity (exercise tolerance).
- Evaluation of the efficacy of medical and/or surgical treatment for CAD.

Minor Indications of the Exercise ECG Test

- Assessment of the nature of certain (exercise-induced) cardiac arrhythmias and chronotropic incompetence.
- Evaluation of exercise-related symptoms.

- Screening purposes (general population, certain occupations, life insurance).
- Rehabilitation of cardiac patients.
- Research purposes.

Contraindications of the Exercise ECG Test

Contraindications can be categorized into absolute versus relative reasons.

Absolute Contraindications

- Acute MI within two days or active unstable angina pectoris.
- Decompensated heart failure (HF).
- Uncontrolled cardiac arrhythmia with hemodynamic compromise.
- Symptomatic severe aortic stenosis.
- Active infective endocarditis.
- Acute pulmonary embolism, pulmonary infarction, or deep vein thrombosis.
- Acute myocarditis or pericarditis.
- Acute aortic syndrome (aortic dissection, intramural hematoma, penetrating ulcer).
- Other acute illness (acute hepatitis, acute renal failure, pneumonia, high fever, etc.).
- Known or suspected obstructive left main coronary artery stenosis.
- Physical or mental disability precluding safe and adequate testing.

Relative Contraindications

- Moderate to severe aortic stenosis with uncertain relation to symptoms.
- Atrial tachyarrhythmias with uncontrolled ventricular rates.

- Acquired advanced or complete heart block.
- Hypertrophic obstructive cardiomyopathy with severe resting gradient.
- Recent stroke or transient ischemic attack.
- Resting hypertension with systolic or diastolic BPs >200/110 mmHg.
- Uncorrected medical conditions such as significant anemia, electrolyte imbalance, and hyperthyroidism.

Interpretations of the ECG Stress Test

As will be discussed further in Chapter 14, several ECG and clinical criteria are examined when interpreting an ECG stress test. With regard to the ECG response itself:

- The most reliable criterion for an abnormal response is occurrence of horizontal or downsloping ST-segment depression ≥1 mm at 60–80 ms after the J point.
- A less common finding is the occurrence of ST-segment elevation >1.0 mm at 60 ms after the J point in leads without pre-existing Q waves because of prior MI (exceptions: leads aVR, aVL, and V1). In subjects without previous infarction, indicated by absence of Q waves on the resting ECG, ST-segment elevation localizes the site of ischemia (most often due to significant subtotal proximal occlusive CAD). In patients with ST-segment elevation and a prior Q-wave MI, the ST-segment elevation in leads with Q waves is believed to be due to abnormal wall motion in the infarct territory or peri-infarction ischemia.
- Functional ST-segment depression (J-point depression) up to 2 mm is considered to be insignificant unless the depression persists beyond 80 ms, so-called "slow-upsloping ST depression." This degree of upsloping ST-segment depression, however, is considered an "equivocal" response.

- Another purported finding indicative of an abnormal exercise ECG response is inversion of U-waves (rare phenomenon).
- Clinically insignificant ECG findings include phenomenon such as isolated T-wave changes, development of bundle branch block, or peaking of the P-waves during or after exercise.

Factors Influencing the Result: False Positive/Negative Stress ECG Tests (see Chapter 15)

The incidence of false positive or false negative stress ECG test results varies depending upon the diagnostic criteria used, prevalence (pre-test likelihood) of CAD in the population, and several other factors.

False "positive" stress ECG test results are more commonly found in women compared to men due to lower prevalence of CAD. Other conditions associated with false positive test results may include use of medications such as digitalis (less commonly encountered today) and diuretics (rare and only when hypokalemia is present) and with ECG abnormalities which affect repolarization such as left bundle branch block, Wolff-Parkinson-White pattern, left ventricular (LV) hypertrophy, and resting ST/T abnormality.

False "negative" results are most commonly encountered when submaximal exercise stress is performed, with borderline significant coronary artery narrowing or in the presence of less extensive CAD (especially single-vessel left circumflex CAD). Use of anti-anginal medications at the time of testing may also lead to a false "negative" result.

Clinical Values of the Exercise ECG Test

In order to better understand the clinical value of the exercise ECG test it is important to be familiar with the concepts of test sensitivity, specificity, predictive value, and prevalence of disease.

Sensitivity of a test refers to the percentage of patients with disease who are detected correctly (abnormal test result).

Sensitivity = True positives / True positives + False negatives

Specificity of a test is the ability of a negative test to identify those who do not have disease.

Specificity = True negatives / True negatives + False positives.

Based on the results of a large meta-analysis of the exercise ECG stress test, the test performance for the detection of angiographically-significant CAD revealed a mean test sensitivity of 68% and a mean test specificity of 77%. In this analysis, a wide range of sensitivities and specificities was found, likely due to the presence of multiple factors including definitions of what constituted significant CAD, disease prevalence in the various populations studied, and conditions that can lead to false positive or negative results as listed above.

Predictive values help to define the diagnostic value of a test; they are highly influenced by the prevalence of disease in the population being tested.

Positive predictive value of an abnormal ("positive") test is the percentage of abnormal tests which indicate presence of disease.

Positive predictive value = True positives / True positives + False positives.

Negative predictive value represents the percentage of normal ("negative") tests that indicate lack of disease.

Negative predictive value = True negatives / True negatives + false negatives.

Bayes' theorem relates that the probability of having disease following performance of the test equals the product of the pre-test probability of having the disease and the probability that the test provided a true result (post-test probability). A test would have a greater positive predictive value and lower negative predictive value when used in a population with a high prevalence of disease. In converse, when used in a population with a lower prevalence of the disease, the same test would be expected to have a higher negative predictive value and lower positive predictive value.

Without doubt, the multistage exercise ECG stress test provides useful information in the evaluation and management of patients with known or suspected CAD in terms of both diagnosis and assessment of functional capacity. When used in a population with an intermediate pre-test likelihood of disease, the predictive value (diagnostic performance) of the test is good. However, the value of the exercise ECG test is limited when dealing with asymptomatic and generally healthy individuals because of the extremely high incidence of false positive test results.

Numerous studies have documented the correlation between the number and location of diseased coronary vessels and the extent and magnitude of ST-segment changes induced by exercise. In general, the presence of ischemia detected during an exercise ECG stress test more often occurs in patients with higher disease prevalence and greater anatomical extent of CAD. Note that while ST-segment depression occurring during an exercise ECG stress test represents the presence of sub-endocardial ischemia; it *does not serve to localize* the anatomical region(s) of ischemia.

Cardiac Arrhythmias and the Exercise ECG Test (Chapter 12)

Various cardiac arrhythmias may be induced or abolished by exercise. Ventricular arrhythmias are seen commonly with exercise in both healthy subjects and in patients with various cardiovascular disorders, particularly CAD.

- CAD may be strongly suspected when serious ventricular arrhythmias (multiform or grouped ventricular premature contractions [VPCs], VT) develop in conjunction with the onset of exercise-induced angina pectoris even in the absence of ST-segment changes.

- Isolated findings of exercise-induced ventricular arrhythmias are not diagnostic of CAD.
- Exercise-induced ventricular arrhythmias may commonly occur in patients with cardiomyopathy or mitral valve prolapse syndrome (MVPS).
- Supraventricular arrhythmias occur less commonly during exercise and their development is not diagnostic of organic heart disease.
- Atrial premature contractions (APCs), with or without grouped beats and short runs of atrial tachycardia (AT), are the most common supraventricular arrhythmias that occur with exercise.

Hemodynamic Responses to Exercise

Monitoring Requirements

- A continuous display of the ECG with periodic print-outs (usually near the end of each stage) is mandatory during the exercise/stress phase and for at least six to eight minutes during the recovery phase for detection of ST-segment changes and cardiac arrhythmias.
- It is essential to measure BP by applying an appropriately-sized cuff to an upper extremity during each stage of stress and for at least six to eight minutes during the recovery phase.
- It is prudent to obtain additional ECG and BP recordings with any change in symptom status, adverse physical signs, and with the occurrence of significant arrhythmias.

Adverse Hemodynamic Responses

- Patients who demonstrate less than expected acceleration of HR (chronotropic incompetence) during a multistage exercise protocol have an increased risk for overt cardiovascular events.

- Some patients with advanced CAD may develop actual slowing of the HR during progressive exercise. This finding is often associated with angina pectoris, but not necessarily with ST-segment shifts.
- A less than expected increment of the sinus rate during exercise may also be a manifestation of sick sinus syndrome.
- Multi-vessel CAD should be suspected when a reproducible and sustained reduction of SBP of ≥10 mmHg occurs during exercise, especially when angina pectoris and/or ST-segment changes coincide. This type of response may occur in approximately 5% of exercise ECG stress tests in a busy stress laboratory. While the majority of such patients are found to have normal LV function at rest, LV dysfunction may have been present at rest or developed with exercise.
- An exaggerated SBP response to exercise is considered to have occurred when maximal value is ≥210 mmHg for men and ≥190 mmHg for women. A rise in DBP during exercise of >10 mmHg above the resting value or an absolute value of 90 mmHg is considered abnormal and could predict increased likelihood of CAD. Recommended relative indications for exercise test termination are SBP of >250 mmHg and/or a DBP >115 mmHg.
- The healthcare professional monitoring the stress test must be able to distinguish pathological responses of HR and BP during exercise stress from similar responses that may occur during the first stage of exercise among normal individuals who are anxious prior to the exercise ECG test.

Complications and Potential Risks (Chapters 12 and 21)

Overall, exercise testing is considered a safe procedure with a low risk of morbidity and mortality: the incidence of an acute coronary event or cardiac death is estimated to be 1/10 000 cases. Nonetheless, associated cardiovascular events such as serious cardiac arrhythmias (particularly ventricular tachyarrhythmias), acute MI, or even cardiac death may occur during or after stress testing. Careful consideration of contraindications should be reviewed prior to testing and all appropriate precautions and monitoring should be taken during and following the stress testing bout to prevent potentially major complications from occurring.

References

Fletcher, G.F., Ades, P.A., Kligfield, P. et al., American Heart Association Exercise, Cardiac Rehabilitation, and Prevention Committee of the Council on Clinical Cardiology, Council on Nutrition, Physical Activity and Metabolism, Council on Cardiovascular and Stroke Nursing, and Council on Epidemiology and Prevention (2013). Exercise standards for testing and training: a scientific statement from the American Heart Association. *Circulation* 128: 873–934.

Gianrossi, R., Detrano, R., Mulvihill, D. et al. (1989). Exercise-induced ST depression in the diagnosis of coronary artery disease. A meta-analysis. *Circulation* 80: 87–98.

Le, V.V., Mitiku, T., Sungar, G. et al. (2008). The blood pressure response to dynamic exercise testing: a systematic review. *Prog. Cardiovasc. Dis.* 51: 135–160.

Myers, J., Arena, R., Franklin, B. et al., American Heart Association Committee on Exercise, Cardiac Rehabilitation, and Prevention of the Council on Clinical Cardiology, the Council on Nutrition, Physical Activity, and Metabolism, and the Council on Cardiovascular Nursing (2009). Recommendations for clinical exercise laboratories: a scientific statement from the American Heart Association. *Circulation* 119: 3144–3161.

Rochmis, P. and Blackburn, H. (1971). Exercise tests. A survey of procedures, safety, and litigation experience in approximately 170,000 tests. *JAMA* 217: 1061–1066.

Rodgers, G.P., Ayanian, J.Z., Balady, G. et al. (2000). American College of Cardiology/American Heart Association clinical competence statement on stress testing: a report of the American College of Cardiology/American Heart Association/American College of Physicians-American Society of Internal Medicine Task Force on Clinical Competence. *Circulation* 102: 1726–1738.

2   Preparations and Precautions

Bryon A. Gentile

Introduction

As with many aspects of diagnostic testing, making the proper preparations and observing appropriate precautions are essential to ensuring patient safety and producing the highest-quality exercise ECG tracings.

Prior to testing, the appropriate personnel must be present. Providers supervising exercise testing must be thoroughly versed in the entire procedure as well as interpretation of the study. Providers should understand the indication for testing in each individual patient and should perform a relevant history and physical examination to identify absolute and relative contraindications to the procedure as well as identify patient characteristics that may reduce the sensitivity and specificity of the examination (medications, left bundle branch block [LBBB], Wolff-Parkinson-White [WPW], etc.).

Proper equipment is essential to produce high-quality ECG tracings. In this endeavor, proper skin preparation, the use of proper electrodes, and the most suitable ECG lead system are needed to detect ST-segment changes in the maximal degree.

Pocket Guide to Stress Testing, Second Edition. Edited by Dennis A. Tighe and Bryon A. Gentile.
© 2020 John Wiley & Sons Ltd. Published 2020 by John Wiley & Sons Ltd.

Preparations and Precautions

Personnel

Appropriate healthcare professionals must be present to supervise the exercise ECG test. This may include a physician, advanced practice provider (nurse practitioner, physician assistants, etc.), or an exercise physiologist. Ultimately the medical director of the exercise laboratory is responsible for the structure and operation of the laboratory. Regardless of the personnel directly monitoring patient exercise, a supervising physician must be readily available for assistance and direction.

In many medical institutions, well-trained cardiac nurses or exercise technicians are available to assist healthcare professionals in the performance of these examinations.

All healthcare professionals should be well versed and have documented completion of an American Heart Association (AHA)-sponsored basic life support (BLS) course. For providers supervising exercise, certification in advanced cardiac life support (ACLS) and emergency cardiac care is mandatory. Requirements for physician competency in data interpretation have been outlined in published guidelines by the American College of Cardiology (ACC)/AHA.

Environment, Equipment, and Medications

The testing environment should be well lighted, kept at a comfortable temperature, and large enough for providers to perform a relevant history and physical examination, in addition to accommodating all necessary equipment, including equipment for providing emergency cardiac care.

Exercise Treadmill

An electrically-driven treadmill is utilized in most laboratories. It should accommodate a variety of body weights up to 350 lbs (157.5 kg). Electronic controls should allow for a range of speeds from 1 to 8 mph (1.6–12.8 kph), and the ability to achieve 20% elevation. An emergency stop button should be readily accessible to both staff and patients. Handrails should be available for safety. However, excessive support during exercise should be discouraged as this decreases the metabolic work done during exercise.

Some laboratories utilize bicycles or arm ergometers as an alternative when patients are unable to exercise on a treadmill.

Medications and Equipment

In rare circumstances, use of emergency equipment may become necessary. The minimum equipment and medications needed in an exercise testing laboratory is listed in Table 2.1. A well-maintained defibrillator should be present in every laboratory without exception.

In some facilities, a comprehensive equipment cart may be located outside the testing area. A clearly defined plan for accessing such equipment in an emergency situation should be established and practiced.

Preparations by and for Patients

Patients should arrive in comfortable clothing with appropriate footwear at least three hours after a light meal. Medications taken with a small amount of water prior to testing is permissible.

Reviewing the Procedure with Patients

The healthcare professional performing the procedure should discuss the entire procedure, in detail, with the patient. Symptoms such as angina or impending syncope should be reviewed prior to exercise and the patient should be instructed to report the onset of such symptoms at once. The patient should be reminded that they may request that exercise stop prematurely whenever necessary.

If the patient is not familiar with the use of a treadmill or bicycle, a brief demonstration is likely to be helpful.

Table 2.1 Emergency equipment, medications, and fluids.

Emergency Equipment

Portable defibrillator

Oxygen (preferably portable)

Oxygen delivery equipment: nasal cannula, venti/non-rebreather masks, etc.

Ventilatory equipment: oral and nasopharyngeal airways, bag-valve-mask respirator

Intubation and suction equipment

Intravenous catheters, syringes, needles, tubing, and infusion pump

Medications

Chewable aspirin

Sublingual nitroglycerin

Adenosine

Atropine

Dobutamine

Vasopressors: epinephrine, dopamine, vasopressin

Chronotropic agents: intravenous metoprolol, diltiazem, and verapamil

Antiarrhythmic agents: amiodarone and lidocaine

Theophylline (for laboratories performing adenosine, dipyridamole, or regadenoson testing)

Medications to treat allergic reactions: epinephrine injector, dexamethasone, diphenhydramine, and albuterol *(for laboratories performing contrast echocardiography and vasodilator testing)*

Intravenous fluids

Normal saline/lactated Ringer's and D5W

Potential complications should be reviewed with patient. Complications such as sudden death, myocardial infarction (MI), or significant arrhythmia requiring hospitalization are generally quoted at a rate of 1-2/10 000.

Informed Consent

Once the procedure has been explained to the patient, the risks, benefits, and alternatives to the procedure should be reviewed with the patient and informed consent should be obtained. Requirements for obtaining informed consent vary internationally. However, many exercise ECG laboratories, particularly in the United States, require obtaining such consent for medico-legal purposes. An example of an informed consent form used for exercise ECG testing can be found in Table 2.2. Other examples of informed consent forms can be found in published recommendations by the AHA.

History Taking and Physical Examination

Although the referring provider has generally obtained a thorough history and physical examination, it remains essential for the provider supervising exercise to obtain a focused history and physical examination to identify contraindications (reviewed separately in Chapter 4) and identify high-risk features in patients. It is also important to identify the patient's index symptoms, including atypical symptoms, such that these can be monitored during testing.

Signs and symptoms that may warrant alterations in plans for stress testing may include:

- *Congestive heart failure* (CHF). Historical features such as orthopnea, paroxysmal nocturnal dyspnea, and exertional dyspnea are suspicious for CHF and signs such as a gallop rhythm, pulmonary rales, cardiomegaly, jugular venous distention, and peripheral edema may yield a diagnosis.

Table 2.2 Sample exercise ECG laboratory consent form.

Procedure: Exercise (stress) ECC testing or Exercise (stress) echocardiogram

Date procedure will be performed:

Attending Physician directing procedure:

Provider performing procedure (if different from Attending Physician):

Signature of provider performing the procedure:

This test is designed to evaluate for the presence of significant heart disease, such as coronary heart disease, and/or evaluate the efficacy of my current therapy, and/or measure my physical fitness for work and/or athletics.

I understand that I will walk on a motor-driven treadmill. During the performance of the exercise ECG test, my electrocardiogram will be monitored and my blood pressure will be measured and recorded at periodic intervals. The exercise will progressively increase according to the standard schedule until I attain a predetermined endpoint corresponding to moderate exercise stress, or become distressed, or develop an abnormal response, whichever occurs first. I understand that I may request that the test be discontinued at any time.

I understand that as with other diagnostics tests, there are potential risks associated with this test. These include falling, weakness, lightheadedness, fainting, chest discomfort, leg cramps, and palpitations. On rare occasions (approximately 2–3/10 000) a heart attack (myocardial infarction [MI]) or sudden death (approximately 1/10 000) may occur. I understand that the exercise laboratory is properly equipped for such situations and that its personnel are trained to administer any emergency care necessary.

Signature of Patient or Authorized Representative:

Signature of Person Witnessing Patient's Signature:

Date:

- *Physical disabilities* may impair the patient's ability to exercise and may warrant conversion to a pharmacological study.
- *Abnormal vital signs*, such as fever, tachy- or bradyarrhythmias, severe hypertension, or respiratory distress.
- *Loud systolic or diastolic murmurs* may indicate significant valvular heart disease such as aortic stenosis, mitral stenosis, or mitral regurgitation.
- *Medications* that may interfere with study interpretation. Digitalis commonly results in ST-segment abnormalities and will reduce the specificity of testing, while beta-blockers and other anti-anginal medications may blunt an ischemic response, reducing the sensitivity in studies performed for the diagnosis of coronary artery disease (CAD).

Ancillary Testing

Review of ancillary testing that has previously been performed may be helpful in identifying contraindications to exercise or high-risk features.

- *Electrocardiogram*. Some patients will have a prior ECG available. Review of this study may demonstrate the need for myocardial imaging such as left ventricular hypertrophy (LVH) with repolarization abnormalities, WPW syndrome, LBBB, or ventricular pacing. Comparison of a prior ECG with the one performed prior to exercise may demonstrate evidence of active ischemia or interval infarct.
- *Electrolyte imbalances* (reviewed separate in Chapter 15), may result in false positive tests.
- *Echocardiography* may demonstrate evidence of a prior MI manifesting as a wall motion abnormality or uncover valvular heart disease that was previously not suspected on physical examination.

12-Lead Electrocardiogram

Obtaining a standard 12-lead ECG prior to exercise is essential to identify abnormalities that may warrant alterations to the proposed testing.

- Conduction abnormalities such as LBBB, ventricular pacing, LVH with repolarization abnormalities, or WPW syndrome are unlikely provide diagnostic test results without concurrent myocardial imaging.
- Conditions such as atrial fibrillation with rapid ventricular response, supraventricular tachycardia, or ventricular arrhythmias preclude exercise testing.

When a multichannel ECG recorder is available, a complete 12-lead ECG may be obtained instantly at any time during the procedure. In our laboratory a 12-lead ECG is obtained:

- Before and after exercise.
- At the conclusion of each stage of exercise.
- When significant ST depression is noted.
- With symptoms of angina or anginal equivalent.
- When a significant arrhythmia occurs.

Skin Preparation and Electrode Placement

Baseline artifact will affect the interpretation of the exercise ECG. Therefore, proper skin preparation and specially designed electrodes are required to produce high-quality ECG recordings.

Skin Preparation

- If excessive hair is present in the areas where electrodes will be placed, this should be removed. Oil should be removed with an organic solvent and allowed to dry.

- The superficial keratinized layer of epidermis should be removed by gentle skin abrasion with a mild abrasive substance such as fine sandpaper or emery board. Commercially prepared products are also available.
- Excessive debridement should be avoided to prevent local tissue edema and increase resistance of the electrode-skin interface.

Electrodes

- Lightweight silver-silver chloride electrodes are recommended. These minimize the loss of contact that often occurs with motion, particularly during peak exercise.
- Shielded electrode cables attached via a belt mounted hub worn around the waist can also reduce motion artifact, as can securing cables to the chest with tape or other commercially available products.
- Once connected, it is often helpful to simulate walking or gently tapping the electrodes to assess for excessive artifact.

Lead Systems

Proper selection of lead systems is important and should meet the requirements set forth by the AHA. While use of a multichannel lead system capable of obtaining a simultaneous 12-lead ECG is highly recommended, single-channel and other multichannel lead systems remain available.

Single-Channel Systems

- When a single-channel ECG recorder is available, various modified bipolar lead V5 positions are the best selection. The positive electrode is placed in the fifth left intercostal space at the anterior axillary line; the negative electrode can be placed in a variety of positions, including the forehead (CH_3), right infraclavicular area (CS_5), left fifth intercostal space (CC_5), or the back (CA_5).

- Lead CM_5 is the most popular among the modified bipolar lead V_5 and exhibits high sensitivity. When lead CM_5 does not record the highest R-wave amplitude, the electrode placement in some patients may be modified to register the tallest R-wave amplitude.

Multichannel Systems Other than 12 Lead

- When a two-channel recorder is available, lead CM_5 and lead II (or aVF) should be considered.
- When a three-channel recorder is available, the addition of modified lead V3 should be considered.

Blood Pressure (BP) Monitoring

It is essential to measure and record BP during and after exercise as the so-called double product (systolic blood pressure [SBP] multiplied by the heart rate [HR]) is an excellent index of myocardial oxygen consumption. Furthermore, the development of hypotension or a flat BP response during exercise are suggestive of CAD and/or left ventricular (LV) dysfunction.

- BP can be challenging to measuring during exercise. Manual auscultation with an appropriately fitted cuff is recommended. If automated systems are utilized, they should be validated against manual recordings prior to routine use.
- BP should be monitored during the last 30 seconds of each stage for interval protocols or the last 30 seconds of each 2-minute interval for ramping protocols.
- BP should also be monitored in the post-exercise recovery period until it returns to near-baseline level.

Premature Test Termination

The most important role of the healthcare professional supervising exercise is to identify conditions that warrant premature test termination and administer treatment when necessary.

- Symptoms such as severe chest pain, impending syncope or fall, and signs such as cyanosis, pallor, or hypotension warrant discontinuation of exercise.
- Arrhythmias such as ventricular tachycardia (VT), ischemic ECG changes such as marked horizontal or downsloping ST-segment depression of ≥2 mm (especially if symptoms or abnormal hemodynamic responses are also present) should prompt premature test termination.

Administration of Treatment as Needed

Supervising health care professionals must determine whether immediate treatment is needed.

- Use of sublingual nitroglycerin is not uncommon for exercise-induced angina.
- Nasal oxygen may be required to treat hypoxia.
- Occasionally, antiarrhythmic drugs such as amiodarone or adenosine are needed for ventricular or supraventricular arrhythmias, respectively.
- On rare occasions, hospitalization may be required if patients develop an acute coronary syndrome, significant arrhythmia, or have prolonged abnormality of the ECG or vital signs after exercise.
- Rarely, ACLS algorithms will need to be employed in the setting of a cardiac emergency.

Follow-up care and management will be addressed in detail in Chapter 17.1

Summary

- A proper testing environment, with fully functioning equipment and immediate access to appropriate medications, is essential for providing safe and effective exercise stress testing.
- Appropriate healthcare professionals, trained in BLS and ACLS, must be present to supervise the exercise ECG test. This may include a physician, advanced practice provider, or exercise physiologist. A qualified physician directing exercise testing must be immediately available for assistance and direction as needed.
- Emergency equipment and medications (Table 2.1), including a defibrillator, must be present.
- The entire procedure should be discussed with the patient prior to exercise, including a demonstration of treadmill use if needed.
- After a discussion of potential complications, including sudden death, MI, and significant arrhythmias, informed consent should be obtained and documented.
- Obtaining a focused history and physical examination is essential to identify index symptoms, potential contraindications, and high-risk features that would impact test performance.
- Review of ancillary testing can be helpful in identifying conditions that may result in warrant the addition of imaging.
- Obtaining a standard 12-lead ECG is mandatory prior to and after exercise. It is helpful to compare this with a prior ECG as this may demonstrate interval infarction or active ischemia.
- Use of high-quality electrodes, cables, and a multichannel lead system capable of obtaining full 12-lead ECGs is recommended.
- BP should be monitored during the last 30 seconds of each stage for interval protocols or the last 30 seconds of each 2-minute interval for ramping protocols.
- Healthcare professions supervising exercise must be capable of identifying conditions that warrant premature test termination and administer treatment as needed.

References

Fletcher, G.F., Ades, P.A., Kligfield, P. et al., on behalf of the American Heart Association Exercise, Cardiac Rehabilitation, and Prevention Committee of the Council on Clinical Cardiology, Council on Nutrition, Physical Activity and Metabolism, Council on Cardiovascular and Stroke Nursing, and Council on Epidemiology and Prevention (2013). Exercise standards for testing and training: A scientific statement from the American Heart Association. *Circulation* 128: 873–934.

Gibbons, R.J., Balady, G.J., Bricker, J.T. et al. (2002). ACC/AHA 2002 guideline update for exercise testing: a report of the American College of Cardiology/American Heart Association task force on practice guidelines (committee on exercise testing). *Circulation* 106: 1883–1892.

Kligfield, P., Gettes, L.S., Bailey, J.J. et al. (2007). Recommendations for the standardization and interpretation of the electrocardiogram: part l: the electrocardiogram and its technology: a scientific statement from the American Heart Association Electrocardiography and Arrhythmias Committee, Council on Clinical Cardiology; the American College of Cardiology Foundation; and the Heart Rhythm Society. *Circulation* 115: 1306–1324.

Myers, J., Arena, R., Franklin, B. et al., American Heart Association Committee on Exercise, Cardiac Rehabilitation, and Prevention of the Council on Clinical Cardiology, the Council on Nutrition, Physical Activity, and Metabolism, and the Council on Cardiovascular Nursing (2009). Recommendations for clinical exercise laboratories: a scientific statement from the American Heart Association. *Circulation* 119: 3144–3161.

Rodgers, G.P., Ayanian, J.Z., Balady, G. et al. (2000). American College of Cardiology/American Heart Association clinical competence statement on stress testing. *Circulation* 102: 1726–1738.

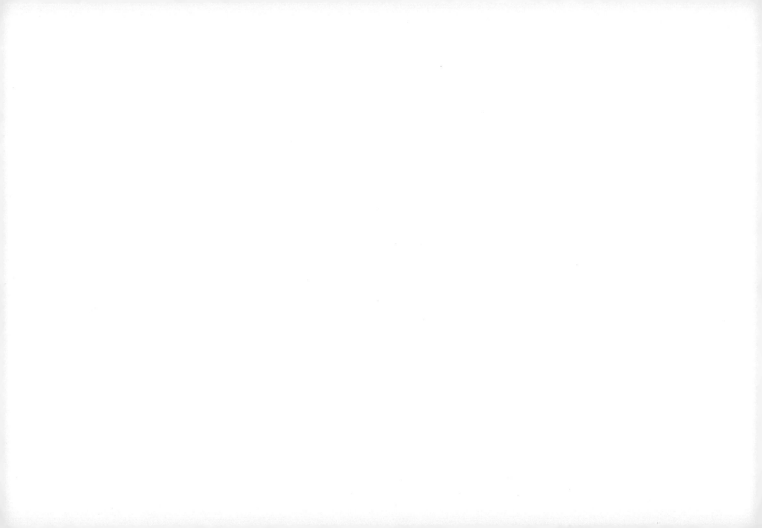

3 Indications

Bryon A. Gentile

Introduction

As with any procedure, the objectives of the study should be clearly identified prior to testing. This chapter reviews the most common indications for exercise ECG stress testing (Table 3.1).

By far the most common indication for exercise ECG stress testing is the evaluation of chest pain syndromes (or symptom equivalents) and diagnosis of obstructive coronary artery disease (CAD). Exercise stress testing also provides important insight into the functional capacity of patients and, with the addition of prognostic scoring such as the Duke treadmill score (DTS), can provide a prediction of future cardiovascular events and all-cause mortality.

Other indications for exercise ECG testing include evaluation chronotropic competence, assessment for exercise-induced arrhythmias, as well as response to device-based therapy. Additionally, exercise ECG testing can be used to evaluate a patient's response to therapeutic interventions, including pharmacotherapy.

Less common indications include screening purposes for specific activities or occupations.

Pocket Guide to Stress Testing, Second Edition. Edited by Dennis A. Tighe and Bryon A. Gentile.
© 2020 John Wiley & Sons Ltd. Published 2020 by John Wiley & Sons Ltd.

Table 3.1 Indications for exercise ECG testing.

Diagnostic purposes

    Assessment of chest pain syndromes

    Diagnosis of coronary artery disease (CAD)

    Diagnosis of exercise-induced arrhythmias

Evaluation purposes

    Exercise capacity and functional classification

    Efficacy of medical therapy for CAD (anti-anginal therapy, etc.)

    Efficacy of revascularization therapy for CAD

    Prognostication by aerobic exercise capacity

    Evaluation of dyspnea

Rehabilitation purposes

    Cardiac and vascular rehabilitation

Screening purposes

    Life insurance/health insurance

    Risk stratification in certain occupations (e.g. pilots)

Indications

Diagnostic Purposes

The most important indication for exercise stress testing is for the evaluation of chest pain syndromes and diagnosis of obstructive CAD.

Exercise stress testing provides objective evidence of CAD that has been suspected or clinically diagnosed. Typical angina pectoris exhibits reproducibility with exercise at similar workloads, while atypical or non-cardiac chest pain is usually not reproducible by repeated exercise.

The reliability of ST-segment depression for the diagnosis of CAD is influenced by factors including the magnitude and morphology of the ST-segment depression, its onset in relation to the exercise workload, and the duration of the ischemic ECG changes during the recovery period.

As with any diagnostic test, the sensitivity and specificity of the exercise ECG will vary with the diagnostic criteria used for a positive test, the characteristics of the population under study, as well as the definition of "hemodynamically significant" CAD as defined by coronary angiography.

Exercise testing can be helpful in the diagnosis of exercise-induced arrhythmias. Arrhythmias may be provoked or suppressed by exercise in healthy patients as well as in patients with CAD. Ventricular arrhythmias provoked by minimal exercise are uncommon in healthy individuals, while the development of ventricular arrhythmias such as multifocal ventricular premature contractions (VPCs), grouped VPCs, or ventricular tachycardia (VT) are highly suggestive of advanced CAD and potentially left ventricular (LV) dysfunction.

Horizontal or downsloping ST-segment depression of 1 mm or greater is generally accepted as the marker for the diagnosis of CAD by exercise ECG, provided that factors such as non-specific ST abnormalities ($\geq 0.5-1.0$ mm

ST-segment depression), left ventricular hypertrophy (LVH) with repolarization abnormalities, left bundle branch block (LBBB), ventricular pacing, digitalis use/effect, or Wolff-Parkinson-White (WPW) pattern have been excluded.

A meta-analysis reviewing 147 studies evaluating the exercise ECG test for the detection of CAD, found a mean sensitivity of 68% and mean specificity of 77%. Sensitivity is highest for patients with three-vessel CAD and is progressively reduced for those with two-vessel and single-vessel CAD.

Evaluation Purposes

In addition to its diagnostic uses, exercise ECG stress testing provides important information for evaluation purposes.

Commonly, exercise testing allows an assessment of a patient's exercise capacity as expressed as metabolic equivalents (METs). Table 3.2 lists the metabolic costs of many common activities.

Aerobic exercise capacity is an important predictor of adverse events in many patient populations, with studies showing a decrease in both cardiovascular morbidity and all-cause mortality as aerobic capacity increases.

Exercise capacity allows patients to be grouped into functional classifications based on the New York Heart Association (NYHA) functional classification (Table 3.3). Once a functional classification is determined, patients may be instructed to limit their activities to comparable workloads.

In patients with known CAD, exercise testing can determine the workload that precipitates symptoms and/or ECG evidence of myocardial ischemia. Such patients may be instructed to limit their activities or exercise to workloads below this level. Additionally, functional capacity can be altered by medical/surgical therapy and may be reassessed with exercise testing.

Exercise testing may be useful for assessing chronotropic competence in patients with underlying conduction system disease.

Table 3.2 Approximate metabolic costs of activities (includes resting metabolic needs).

Metabolic equivalents (METs)	Activity
1.5–2	Standing
	Walking at 1 mph (1.6 km/h)
2–2.5	Playing cards
	Sewing, knitting
2–3	Walking at 2 mph (3.25 km/h)
	Cycling at 5 mph (8 km/h)
2.5–4	Billiards
	Bowling
	Shuffleboard
	Golf (power cart)
	Playing piano and many musical instruments
3–4	Walking at 2.5 mph (4 km/h)
	Cycling at 6 mph (10 km/h)
4–5	Leisure volleyball
	Golf (pull cart)
	Badminton
	Pushing light lawn mower

(*Continued*)

Table 3.2 (Continued)

Metabolic equivalents (METs)	Activity
	Walking at 3 mph (5 km/h)
	Cycling at 8 mph (13 km/h)
	Table tennis
5–6	Golf (carrying clubs)
	Dancing
	Doubles tennis
	Raking leaves
	Walking at 3.5 mph (5.5 km/h)
	Cycling at 10 mph (16 km/h)
	Ice or roller skating at 9 mph (15 km/h)
6–7	Shoveling for 10 min, 10 lbs (4.5 kg)
	Walking at 5 mph (8 km/h)
	Cycling at 11 mph (17.5 km/h)
	Singles tennis
	Splitting wood
	Manual lawn mowing
	Light downhill skiing
7–8	Jogging at 5 mph
	Cycling at 12 mph (19 km/h)

Table 3.2 (Continued)

Metabolic equivalents (METs)	Activity
8–10	Vigorous downhill skiing
	Basketball
	Ice hockey
	Mountain climbing
	Touch football
	Running at 5.5 mph (9 km/h)
	Cycling at 13 mph (21 km/h)
10–11	Vigorous basketball
	Handball
	Fencing
10+	Shoveling for 10 min, 16 lbs (7.5 kg)
	Running at 6 mph = 10 METs
	Running at 7 mph = 11.5 METs
	Running at 8 mph = 13.5 METs
	Running at 9 mph = 15 METs
	Running at 10 mph = 17 METs

1 MET = 3.5 mlO_2/min/kg for a 70 kg man

Table 3.3 New York Heart Association (NYHA) functional classification and corresponding anticipated workloads.

Class	Workload
I	6–10 METs (metabolic equivalents)
II	4–6 METs
III	2–3 METs
IV	1 MET

The exercise ECG stress test also provides valuable information on healthy individuals who plan to engage in strenuous work, competitive sports, or intense exercise programs. Sedentary individuals who are otherwise healthy can perform workloads in excess of 10–11 METs, while conditioned individuals may be able to perform exercise workloads beyond 16 METs.

Rehabilitation Purposes and Preventative Measures

Exercise ECG stress testing is a useful tool for rehabilitation purposes and preventative measures. Properly designed exercise programs can improve the functional capacity of patients with prior myocardial infarction (MI) or heart failure (HF). This is particularly important in certain occupations with strenuous physical activity.

Screening Purposes

Exercise response and functional capacity, as determined by exercise stress testing, may be required to determine if a subject has the physical working capability to engage in strenuous activities or occupations. It may also be used to screen for occult CAD or high-risk features in persons in specific occupations (e.g. airline pilots).

Exercise ECG stress testing may be used for insurance purposes or in some cases as part of a pre-employment physical examination.

Summary

- Indications and objectives for stress testing must be identified prior to commencing exercise.
- The most common indication for exercise ECG stress testing is the evaluation of chest pain syndromes and the diagnosis of obstructive CAD.
- Exercise ECG stress testing can be valuable for the assessment for exercise-induced arrhythmias.
- Exercise capacity, expressed in METs, and functional classification can be derived from exercise testing and provide guidance for home and occupational activities.
- Prognostication with exercise ECG testing is possible with both cardiovascular morbidity and all-cause mortality decreasing as aerobic capacity increases.
- In patients with known CAD, exercise testing can be used to develop an exercise prescription to avoid workloads provoking ischemia as well as to assess the response to medical and surgical interventions.
- Less commonly, exercise ECG testing can be used to assess the chronotropic competence of patients with underlying conductive system disease.
- Rarely, exercise ECG testing can be used for screening purposes prior to commencement of strenuous activities or occupations. It may also be used to screen for occult CAD or high-risk features in persons in specific occupations.

References

Fletcher, G.F., Ades, P.A., Kligfield, P. et al., on behalf of the American Heart Association Exercise, Cardiac Rehabilitation, and Prevention Committee of the Council on Clinical Cardiology, Council on Nutrition, Physical Activity and Metabolism, Council on Cardiovascular and Stroke Nursing, and Council on Epidemiology and Prevention (2013). Exercise standards for testing and training: a scientific statement from the American Heart Association. *Circulation* 128: 873–934.

Gianrossi, R., Detrano, R., Mulvihill, D. et al. (1989). Exercise-induced ST depression in the diagnosis of coronary artery disease. A meta-analysis. *Circulation* 80: 87–98.

4 Contraindications to Stress Testing

Bryon A. Gentile

Introduction

Exercise stress testing is safe and associated with low morbidity and mortality when performed in appropriate clinical situations. When proper precautions and preparations (Chapter 2) are followed and contraindications have been carefully considered, the risk of complications can be minimized. Major complications include death, acute myocardial infarction (MI), and serious ventricular arrhythmias.

A study from the VA healthcare system with over 60 000 exercise-based tests performed, reported a major complication rate of 1.2 per 10 000 tests with no deaths reported.

Table 4.1 summarizes the absolute and relative contraindications to exercise stress testing.

After reviewing the indications and contraindications to exercise testing it is essential to review a patient's ancillary testing to identify conditions that are likely to yield false positive results or would benefit from the concurrent imaging. Table 4.2 lists such conditions.

Table 4.1 Absolute and relative contraindications to exercise testing.

Absolute contraindications
Acute myocardial infarction within two days
Unstable angina pectoris
Arrhythmia with hemodynamic compromise
Acute myocarditis, pericarditis, or endocarditis
Severe symptomatic aortic stenosis
Decompensated heart failure, cardiogenic shock
Acute aortic dissection
Pulmonary embolism or infarction
Disabilities that preclude safe testing
Relative contraindications
Known obstructive left main coronary stenosis
Moderate to severe aortic stenosis with unclear symptoms
Acquired advanced or complete heart block
Tachyarrhythmias with controlled ventricular rates
Hypertrophic obstructive cardiomyopathy with severe gradient
Resting hypertension with BP greater than 200/110 mmHg
Mental impairment, inability to cooperate, recent stroke or transient ischemic attack
Uncorrected co-morbid conditions (anemia, electrolytes, etc.)

Table 4.2 Conditions known to interfere with ECG interpretation.

Medications and electrolyte abnormalities
- Digoxin use
- Hypokalemia

Cardiac disorders
- Congenital or valvular heart disease
- Cardiomyopathies

Preexisting ECG abnormalities
- Left bundle branch block
- Left ventricular hypertrophy
- Wolff-Parkinson-White pattern/syndrome

Absolute Contraindications

Acute Coronary Syndromes

Acute Myocardial Infarction

Acute MI, within the first 48 hours, is an absolute contraindication to exercise ECG testing due to the risk of life-threating ventricular arrhythmias and worsening infarction. This is particularly true among patients who have not undergone revascularization. If patients admitted with MI are to undergo exercise ECG testing after 48 hours, an appropriate post-MI exercise ECG protocol (Chapter 10) should be followed.

Unstable Angina

Patients with unstable or crescendo angina should not undergo exercise ECG testing due to the risk of MI and life-threatening ventricular arrhythmias that can be provoked with exercise. Following medical stabilization, such patients may become candidates for exercise ECG stress testing (see Chapter 10).

Hemodynamically Significant Arrhythmias

Exercise ECG testing is contraindicated in patients with cardiac arrhythmias such as ventricular tachycardia (VT), uncontrolled atrial dysrhythmias, or acquired advanced/complete atrioventricular (AV) block. Exercise ECG testing can be helpful in the assessment of patients with congenital complete AV block (see Chapter 16).

Acute Myocarditis, Pericarditis, and Endocarditis

Patients with clinical suspicion for acute myocarditis, pericarditis, or endocarditis should not undergo exercise testing due to risk of developing hemodynamically unstable arrhythmias such as VT or ventricular fibrillation.

Symptomatic Severe Aortic Stenosis

Exercise testing yields little information in patients with known symptomatic severe aortic stenosis and should not be performed due to risk of syncope, life-threatening ventricular arrhythmia, or sudden death. With proper preparations (Chapter 2), this can be elucidated by a focused physical examination prior to exercise which may demonstrate a loud systolic ejection murmur obscuring the second heart sound.

Acute Decompensated Heart Failure and Cardiogenic Shock

Exercise testing in patients with acute decompensated HF and cardiogenic shock is contraindicated, as the risks of further decompensation are substantial.

Acute Pulmonary Embolism/Infarction

A focused history and physical examination, combined with persistent sinus tachycardia, may raise a high clinical suspicion of pulmonary embolism. This condition precludes exercise ECG testing due to the risk of malignant arrhythmias and decompensation.

Acute Aortic Dissection

Exercise testing should not be performed in patients with acute aortic dissection as exercise is likely to result in elevations in BP and HR, and potentially propagation of the dissection.

Disabilities Precluding Safe Testing

If patients are unable to safely walk on a treadmill due to physical or mental disabilities, exercise testing should not be performed due to the risk of injury.

Relative Contraindications

Known Left Main Coronary Stenosis

Left main coronary artery stenosis places a large territory of myocardium at risk of ischemia during stress testing. As a result, the risk of complications such as MI, ventricular arrhythmias, and sudden death are increased.

Moderate to Severe Aortic Stenosis and Hypertrophic Obstructive Cardiomyopathy

Exercise testing can help elucidate symptoms in asymptomatic subjects with moderate to severe aortic stenosis and help assess hemodynamic response in patients with obstructive cardiomyopathy, but carries a risk of syncope, ventricular arrhythmias, or even sudden death. If exercise testing is to be pursued, these risks should be carefully reviewed with patients. In our institution, venous access with a peripheral IV is established prior to exercise testing to aid with resuscitative measures in the event of a complication. A physician should directly supervise exercise ECG testing in these patients.

Acquired Advanced or Complete Heart Block

Exercise testing can be useful in patients with advanced or complete heart block to determine chronotropic competence and help guide decisions regarding pacemaker placement. It also carries the risk of syncope and decompensation, and care must be taken to prevent injury in such an event.

Tachyarrhythmias with Controlled Ventricular Rates

Tachyarrhythmias such as atrial fibrillation or multifocal atrial tachycardia can result in uncontrolled (rapid) ventricular response and as such should be managed carefully if referral for exercise testing is considered. Multifocal atrial tachycardia is commonly seen in subjects with underlying lung disease, and as a result, such patients may be at increased risk for worsening hypoxia with exercise testing.

Resting Hypertension (BP >200/110 mmHg)

Pre-existing systemic hypertension will likely be exaggerated during exercise testing and therefore significant resting hypertension is a relative contraindication to exercise testing. In general, exercise should be terminated if systolic blood pressure (SBP) exceeds 250 mmHg and/or diastolic blood pressure (DBP) exceeds 115 mmHg.

Mental Impairment, Inability to Cooperate, or Recent Stroke/TIA

Patient who are unable to cooperate with testing instructions are at risk of injury during exercise stress testing and therefore risks and benefits should carefully be considered. Patients with recent stroke/TIA may have weakness that could increase risk of injury.

Uncorrected Comorbid Conditions

Severe anemia can exacerbate myocardial ischemia. Electrolyte imbalances such as hypokalemia and medication effects from agents such as digoxin can result in false positive testing, while anti-anginal agents such as use of beta-blockers, nitrates, and calcium channel blockers can result in false negative exercise ECG tests.

Summary

- Understanding of and assessment for contraindications to stress testing is as important as understanding testing indications
- With proper precautions, preparations, and review of potential contraindications, complications of exercise ECG stress testing can be avoided.
- Table 4.1 lists absolute and relative contraindications to exercise testing.
- Table 4.2 lists conditions known to interfere with the interpretation of the exercise ECG test.

References

Fletcher, G.F., Ades, P.A., Kligfield, P. et al., on behalf of the American Heart Association Exercise, Cardiac Rehabilitation, and Prevention Committee of the Council on Clinical Cardiology, Council on Nutrition, Physical Activity and Metabolism, Council on Cardiovascular and Stroke Nursing, and Council on Epidemiology and Prevention (2013). Exercise standards for testing and training: a scientific statement from the American Heart Association. *Circulation* 128: 873–934.

Myers, J., Voodi, L., Umann, T., and Froelicher, V.F. (2000). A survey of exercise testing: methods, utilization, interpretation, and safety in the VAHCS. *J. Cardpulm. Rehabil.* 20: 251–258.

5   Exercise Stress ECG Test Protocols

Bryon A. Gentile and Dennis A. Tighe

Introduction

Multiple protocols for exercise ECG stress testing exist; the suitability of each varies according to the objectives of the test and patient characteristics. For example, a vigorous exercise protocol may be suitable for screening purposes among healthy individuals while a milder protocol may be reserved for patients whom have recently suffered an acute coronary syndrome (ACS). General testing procedures and exercise protocols will be reviewed in this chapter. Protocols for pharmacological testing will be reviewed in Chapter 8 and pediatric exercise ECG testing protocols are found in Chapter 16. A complete listing and details of the various protocols can be found in the American College of Sports Medicine's *Guidelines for Exercise Testing and Prescription*.

General Testing Procedures

Patient Instructions and Preparations

When an individual is scheduled for exercise ECG stress testing, patients should be given brief instructions about the test and its conduct (see Chapter 22). In some institutions pamphlets or booklets may be given out at the time of scheduling. In general, we recommend that patients arrive in comfortable clothing and appropriate footwear at least three hours after a light meal. We recommend that medications be continued unless otherwise directed by the referring healthcare provider. If patients are taking anti-anginal medications such as beta-blockers, calcium channel blockers, or long-acting nitrates, we recommend that they consult with their referring provider for specific instructions prior to testing.

On arrival in the exercise laboratory we perform a focused history and physical examination as outlined in Chapter 2. We identify the objectives of the test and review potential contraindications. After reviewing testing, risks, and obtaining an informed consent, the appropriate testing protocol is selected, and exercise is commenced.

Parameters to Be Observed and Assessed

Various parameters must be observed and assessed during and after exercise (Table 5.1). ECG changes, such as ST-segment deviation, blood pressure (BP), and heart rate (HR) changes, must be carefully monitored in conjunction with an assessment of symptoms and physical findings. Exercise capacity can be determined based on the workload achieved. In a similar fashion, the efficacy of medical and/or surgical therapy can be assessed.

Table 5.1 Parameters to be observed and assessed during testing.

ECG changes

ST-segment alterations

    Elevation or depression

    Type and magnitude of depression

    Exercise time and heart rate (HR) at onset

    Post-exercise duration

Arrhythmias

    Mechanisms (origin, type, frequency)

    Relationship to exercise, HR, ST-segment changes, symptoms

Other findings

    Inverted U-waves

    R-wave amplitude

Hemodynamic response

    Blood pressure (BP) and HR changes

    Post-exercise HR recovery

Symptoms and signs

    Onset of symptoms

    Character of symptoms

    Relationship to exercise

    Reproducibility

    Relationship to other findings (e.g. ST-segment, HR and/or BP change)

    S3-S4, murmurs, rales

Miscellaneous

    Assessment of functional capacity (exercise duration)

Exercise Endpoints

It is essential to establish endpoints for exercise. For most indications, exercise should be symptom-limited; HR-limited exercise, terminating testing when 85% of age-predicted maximal HR is achieved, in general, should not be the primary endpoint. In our laboratory, exercise testing is symptom-limited unless specific endpoints are reached (Table 5.2).

Absolute Indications

- When a patient requests the premature termination of exercise testing due to symptoms, testing should stop and the parameters listed in Table 5.1 should be carefully evaluated.
- ST-segment elevation (>1.0 mm) in leads without preexisting Q waves due to prior myocardial infarction (MI) (other than leads aVR, aVL, and V1).
- Abnormal hemodynamic responses, such as hypotension (drop in systolic blood pressure (SBP) by ≥10 mmHg) or bradycardia when accompanied by other evidence of ischemia.
- Exercise should be terminated if the patient develops significant symptoms or signs such as moderate to severe angina, signs of malperfusion (cyanosis or pallor), central nervous system symptoms (ataxia, dizziness, feeling of impending syncope), severe dyspnea, or visual or gait disturbances.
- Testing should be prematurely stopped if the patient develops significant cardiac arrhythmias such as ventricular tachycardia (VT) or ventricular fibrillation or supraventricular tachycardia (SVT) with hemodynamic alteration.
- Acute MI is an absolute indication for test discontinuation.
- Exercise should be discontinued in the event of equipment or testing malfunction.

Relative Indications

- If patient develops significant symptoms, the supervising healthcare professional must determine whether exercise can continue. The most common causes for premature termination are fatigue, dyspnea, leg weakness, and chest pain.

Table 5.2 Indications for terminating exercise testing.

Absolute indications

ST-segment elevation (>1.0 mm) in leads without preexisting Q waves because of prior myocardial infarction (MI) (excluding leads aVR, aVL, and V1)

Drop in blood pressure (BP) and/or heart rate (HR) despite increasing workloads

Moderate to severe angina

CNS symptoms (ataxia, dizziness, near syncope)

Evidence of poor perfusion (cyanosis or pallor)

Sustained ventricular tachycardia (VT) or other arrhythmias such as second- or third-degree heart block

Patient request

Equipment or testing malfunction

Acute MI

Relative indications

Marked ST-segment displacement (horizontal or downsloping ST depression >2 mm measured 60–80 ms after the J point)

Drop in systolic blood pressure (SBP) >10 mmHg despite an increase in workload in the absence of other evidence of ischemia

Increasing chest pain, dyspnea, weakness, fatigue or claudication

Arrhythmias other than sustained VT, including multifocal ectopy, ventricular triplets, SVT, and bradyarrhythmias

Exaggerated hypertensive response (SBP >250 mmHg and/or diastolic blood pressure (DBP) >115 mmHg).

Development of left bundle branch block (LBBB) than cannot be distinguished from VT

- Marked ST-segment displacement (horizontal or downsloping of >2 mm, measured 60–80 ms after the J point in a patient with suspected ischemia).
- Drop in SBP >10 mmHg despite an increase in workload in the absence of other evidence of ischemia.
- Exaggerated hypertensive response (SBP >250 mmHg and/or diastolic blood pressure (DBP) >115 mmHg).
- Arrhythmias other than sustained VT, including multifocal ectopy, ventricular triplets, SVT, and bradyarrhythmias as they have the potential to become more complex or interfere with hemodynamic stability.
- Development of bundle branch block/conduction delay that cannot be immediately distinguished from VT.

Exercise ECG Testing Protocols

A number of exercise protocols are available for use in the clinical exercise laboratory. The suitability of each protocol varies according to the objectives of testing and patient characteristics. The ideal exercise ECG protocol includes:

- An initial workload within the individual's anticipated physical working capacity.
- Workloads increased gradually and maintained for a duration sufficient enough to achieve a near steady state.
- Exercise duration of 8–12 minutes.
- Workload that does not result in excessive mental or physical stress.
- Allows continuous ECG monitoring.

Bruce Protocol

The Bruce protocol (Table 5.3) is one of the most popular protocols utilized in exercise laboratories. The protocol is comprised of seven stages where speed and grade are increased at three-minute intervals. The Bruce protocol has

Table 5.3 Bruce protocol.

Stage	Speed (mph)	Grade (%)	Duration (min)	Metabolic equivalents (METs)	Total elapsed time (min)
1	1.7	10	3	4	3
2	2.5	12	3	6–7	6
3	3.4	14	3	8–9	9
4	4.2	16	3	15–16	12
5	5.0	18	3	21	15
6	5.5	20	3	–	18
7	6.0	22	3	–	21

the advantages of being relatively short in duration and extensive validation. The vigorous nature of this protocol, characterized by large increases in workload at each stage, may be unsuitable for some cardiac or elderly patients (use of the modified Bruce protocol may be a suitable alternative).

Modified Bruce Protocol

Some patients are unable to begin at the workload of the first stage of Bruce protocol. As such, the Modified Bruce protocol (Table 5.4) was developed, with the first two stages performed at 1.7 mph with a 0 and 5% grade, respectively. This may be helpful in elderly or sedentary patients.

Table 5.4 Modified Bruce protocol.

Stage	Speed (mph)	Grade (%)	Duration (min)	Metabolic equivalents (METs)	Total elapsed time (min)
0	1.7	0	3	1–2	3
0.5	1.7	5	3	3–4	6
1	1.7	10	3	4	9
2	2.5	12	3	6–7	12
3	3.4	14	3	8–9	15
4	4.2	16	3	15–16	18
5	5.0	18	3	21	21
6	5.5	20	3	–	24
7	6	22	3	–	27

Naughton Protocol

The Naughton protocol gradually increases workload between stages and may be a good choice for elderly and deconditioned patients. This protocol is often used as the method of exercise stress during cardiopulmonary exercise testing (Chapter 9; Table 5.5).

Table 5.5 Naughton protocol.

Stage	Speed (mph)	Grade (%)	Duration (min)	Metabolic equivalents (METs)	Total elapsed time (min)
1	1	0	2	1–2	2
2	2	0	2	2–3	4
3	2	3.5	2	3–4	6
4	2	7.0	2	4–5	8
5	2	10.5	2	5–6	10
6	2	14.0	2	7–8	12
7	2	17.5	2	8–9	14

Ellestad Protocol

With the Ellestad protocol, the speed is increased progressively every three minutes, from 1.7 to 6.0 mph during six stages. The grade remains constant (10%) for the first four stages, then increases to a 15% grade in stages 5 and 6 (Table 5.6). More ischemic changes can be expected with the Ellestad or Bruce protocol due to their anaerobic nature, but the incidence of false positive results may also be increased.

Table 5.6 Ellestad protocol.

Stage	Speed (mph)	Grade (%)	Duration (min)	Metabolic equivalents (METs)	Total elapsed time (min)
1	1.7	10	3	4	3
2	3	10	2	6–7	5
3	4	10	2	8–9	7
4	5	10	3	10–12	10
5	5	15	2	13–15	12
6	6	15	3	16–20	15

McHenry Protocol

The McHenry protocol uses a warm-up period at 2.0 mph and 3% grade for three minutes. Thereafter, the grade is increased 3% every three minutes, with a constant speed of 3.3 mph during all seven stages (Table 5.7).

Balke and Ware Protocol

The Balke and Ware protocol involves a moderate increase in work rate per stage by maintaining a constant speed (3.3 mph) with an increase in grade by 1% each minute. This protocol may be useful in cardiopulmonary exercise testing, as protocols with large increases in energy requirements between stages have a weaker relationship between measured oxygen consumption and work rate.

Table 5.7 McHenry protocol.

Stage	Speed (mph)	Grade (%)	Duration (min)	Metabolic equivalents (METs)	Total elapsed time (min)
1	2.0	3	3	3–4	3
2	3.3	6	3	6–7	6
3	3.3	9	3	7–8	9
4	3.3	12	3	9	12
5	3.3	15	3	10	15
6	3.3	18	3	11–12	18
7	3.3	21	3	13–14	21

Low-level (Submaximal) Post-Acute Coronary Syndrome Protocols

Exercise testing after ACS is discussed in detail in Chapter 10. In most instances today, the modified Bruce protocol or the Naughton protocol is used (some clinicians prefer a symptom-limited test). A low-level exercise ECG protocol can be used several days post-ACS to identify those stable patients, who have not had reperfusion with primary percutaneous intervention or fibrinolytic therapy or have had incomplete revascularization, who have may have residual myocardial ischemia (high-risk findings with testing). Submaximal protocols are designed to determine functional capacity and identify clinically significant findings, such as signs and symptoms of ischemia or arrhythmias at low workloads, that would prompt performance of coronary angiography prior to discharge. Testing results may be used to guide additional therapies prior to discharge and in the early, post-ACS recovery period. A "negative" submaximal test is usually followed-up with a symptom-limited exercise ECG stress test performed three to six weeks later in clinically stable patients.

In general, end-points for submaximal post-ACS protocols include:

- Peak HR of 120–130 bpm or 70% age-predicted maximal HR.
- Peak workload of five metabolic equivalents (METs).
- ≥2 mm horizontal or downsloping ST-segment depression.
- Exertional hypotension.
- Ventricular ectopy (≥3 consecutive beats).
- Symptoms with exercise (angina pectoris, dyspnea).

Cycle Protocols

In addition to the use of treadmills, protocols have been developed for manually or mechanically-braked cycle ergometers. Cycle ergometry protocols (supine or upright bicycle) may be particularly useful for patients with gait imbalance or difficulty walking on a treadmill; this form of testing is often limited by quadriceps discomfort and fatigue. The cycle ergometer is generally calibrated in watts or kilopond-meters, which can be converted to oxygen uptake and subsequently METs. The cycle ergometer reduces upper body motion, which can limit tracing artifact and simplify BP monitoring. In general, peak workloads with cycle ergometry are about 10–20% lower when compared to treadmill exercise.

Summary

- Preparations are important prior to exercise ECG stress testing. In general, we ask patients to arrive comfortable clothing and appropriate footwear three hours removed from a light meal.
- A focused history and physical examination is recommended. Objectives and potential contraindications of testing should be reviewed. A standard resting 12-lead ECG should be reviewed. Once informed consent has been obtained, exercise can commence.
- Various parameters should be observed and assessed during and after exercise including ECG changes, hemodynamic responses and symptomatic responses to exercise (Table 5.1).
- Endpoints to terminate exercise should be clearly known to the healthcare professional supervising the testing (Table 5.2).
- Various protocols have been developed for exercise ECG stress testing with no single protocol being universally suitable. Use of a particular protocol should include consideration of the objective of the test and patient characteristics. In our institution, the Bruce protocol is most commonly performed, followed by the modified Bruce and Naughton protocols.
- Low-level (submaximal) post-ACS protocols (usually modified Bruce or Naughton protocols) can be used to identify high-risk patients and determine the functional capacity and assess for clinically significant findings such as signs and symptoms of ischemia or arrhythmias at low exercise workloads.
- Cycle ergometer protocols are less commonly used in the United States. In general, peak workloads are about 10–20% lower compared to treadmill exercise.

References

Balady, G.J., Arena, R., Sietsema, K. et al., on behalf of the American Heart Association Exercise, Cardiac Rehabilitation, and Prevention Committee of the Council on Clinical Cardiology, Council on Epidemiology and Prevention; Council on Peripheral Vascular Disease; and Interdisciplinary Council on Quality of Care and Outcomes Research (2010). Clinician's Guide to cardiopulmonary exercise testing in adults: a scientific statement from the American Heart Association. *Circulation* 122: 191–225.

Fletcher, G.F., Ades, P.A., Kligfield, P. et al., on behalf of the American Heart Association Exercise, Cardiac Rehabilitation, and Prevention Committee of the Council on Clinical Cardiology, Council on Nutrition, Physical Activity and Metabolism, Council on Cardiovascular and Stroke Nursing, and Council on Epidemiology and Prevention (2013). Exercise standards for testing and training: a scientific statement from the American Heart Association. *Circulation* 128: 873–934.

Myers, J., Arena, R., Franklin, B. et al., on behalf of the American Heart Association Committee on Exercise, Cardiac Rehabilitation, and Prevention of the Council on Clinical Cardiology, the Council on Nutrition, Physical Activity, and Metabolism, and the Council on Cardiovascular Nursing (2009). Recommendations for clinical exercise laboratories: a scientific statement from the American Heart Association. *Circulation* 119: 3144–3161.

Pescatello, L.S. (2018). *ACSM's Guidelines for Exercise Testing and Prescription*, 10e. Philadelphia: Wolters Kluwer/ Lippincott Williams & Wilkins Health.

6   Stress ECG Testing with Nuclear Myocardial Perfusion Imaging Techniques

Seth T. Dahlberg and Dennis A. Tighe

Introduction

While standard ECG exercise stress testing is widely used for the assessment of suspected or known coronary artery disease (CAD), diagnostic accuracy is limited when pre-existing ECG repolarization or intraventricular conduction abnormalities are present (Table 6.1). In addition, clinical factors can render the standard exercise ECG stress test falsely positive or falsely negative (see Chapter 15). Under these circumstances, stress myocardial perfusion imaging (MPI) provides additional valuable diagnostic information when the exercise ECG test results alone are unreliable for the diagnosis of CAD.

   Radionuclide stress MPI is a nuclear medicine technique that enhances the sensitivity, specificity, and diagnostic accuracy of exercise ECG stress testing in patients with suspected or known cardiac disease. In addition, MPI gives important prognostic information beyond that obtained from the ECG stress test. Single photon MPI using technetium 99 m (^{99m}Tc) labeled sestamibi or tetrofosmin is currently the most widely used radionuclide MPI technique. Thallium-201 (^{201}Tl) is less widely used for MPI due to imaging issues of photon attenuation and scatter

Pocket Guide to Stress Testing, Second Edition. Edited by Dennis A. Tighe and Bryon A. Gentile.
© 2020 John Wiley & Sons Ltd. Published 2020 by John Wiley & Sons Ltd.

Table 6.1 Pre-existing ECG abnormalities affecting repolarization.

- Left bundle branch block (LBBB)
- Right bundle branch block (RBBB) with strain
- Left ventricular hypertrophy (LVH) with strain
- Wolff-Parkinson-White pattern
- Non-specific abnormality of ST-segment (≥0.5 to 1.0 mm ST depression) and T-wave
- Digitalis use/effect
- Mitral valve prolapse syndrome
- Ventricular pacing
- Hypokalemia with ST-segment and T-wave abnormality

as well as the higher radiation dose. While differences in pharmacological properties and kinetics among single photon imaging agents require variation in imaging protocols, the reported diagnostic yields among the clinically available perfusion agents (Table 6.2) are similar. Nuclear perfusion agents are used to assess for the presence of CAD by comparing images obtained at "rest" to those obtained after "stress" (either following standard treadmill exercise or pharmacological stimulation), to assess the vascular distribution and severity of CAD, and to detect viable myocardium.

MPI is typically performed using single photon emission computed tomographic (SPECT) imaging. With this technique photons generated by the injected radioisotope are detected by a single or multicrystal camera. The rotating camera acquires 30–32 projections, each for 20–40 seconds, in a 180° rotation arc around the patient beginning from the 45° right anterior oblique position and preceding to the 45° left posterior oblique position. These multiple projection images are reconstructed into transverse tomographic images and then into standard myocardial

Table 6.2 Properties of clinically used myocardial perfusion agents.

Property	Thallium-201	Technetium 99 m sestamibi or tetrofosmin
Half-life (hr)	73	6
Emitted energy (keV)	69–83 (90%)	140
	167 (10%)	
Dose (mCi)	3.5	25–30 (stress)
		8–12 (rest)
Redistribution	Yes	Minimal
Assess Viability	Yes	Yes
Ability to perform first-pass ejection fraction (EF)	No	Yes
ECG gated imaging	Yes	Yes
Time to complete stress/rest protocol (hr)	3–4	5–6
Clinical experience	++++	++++
Radiation Effective Dose (mSv)	22	9.9–11.3

short-axis (SA), vertical long-axis (VLA), and horizontal long-axis (HLA) images (Figure 6.1). The myocardial distribution of the radiotracer is subsequently analyzed in multiple tomographic slices, permitting assessment of individual coronary vascular territories (Figures 6.2–6.4).

Another technique for radionuclide MPI uses positron emission tomographic (PET) imaging. PET tracers generate positrons which combine with electrons in the myocardial tissue. Each positron/electron pair then generates two

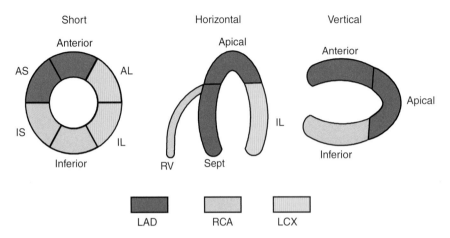

Figure 6.1 Schematic representation of single photon emission computed tomographic (SPECT) images divided into myocardial segments. See text for correlation with distribution of coronary perfusion. AS, anteroseptal; IS, inferoseptal; AL, anterolateral; IL, inferolateral; Sept, septal; RV, right ventricle; LAD, left anterior descending artery; RCA, right coronary artery; LCX, left circumflex artery.

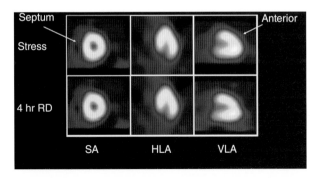

Figure 6.2 Stress and delayed SPECT myocardial perfusion images in the short-axis (SA), horizontal long-axis (HLA), and vertical long-axis (VLA) projections showing normal myocardial perfusion at rest (4 hr RD) and with stress. RD, redistribution.

Figure 6.3 Stress and delayed SPECT myocardial perfusion images in the short-axis (SA), horizontal long-axis (HLA), and vertical long-axis (VLA) projections showing reversible perfusion scan defects consistent with a large area of left anterior descending coronary artery territory ischemia. RD, redistribution.

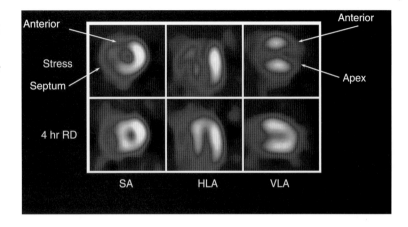

511 keV photons that are imaged with "coincidence detection" using a PET camera with a ring-shaped detector that surrounds the patient. While less widely available than SPECT imaging, PET imaging permits assessment of regional myocardial blood flow, myocardial flow reserve, and myocardial viability or metabolism.

Exercise radionuclide ventriculography (RVG) is an additional nuclear medicine technique which has been used to determine ventricular function in response to stress using planar cardiac imaging. Equilibrium gated imaging uses ^{99m}Tc-labeled red blood cells to determine blood pool activity. After resting images are obtained, exercise (supine bicycle ergometry at our institution) is started. An image is obtained at each stage of exercise for analysis of regional wall motion and ejection fraction (EF). A normal response to progressive exercise is a $\geq 5\%$ increase in EF compared to the resting value without the development of a new wall motion abnormality. Stress RVG imaging can

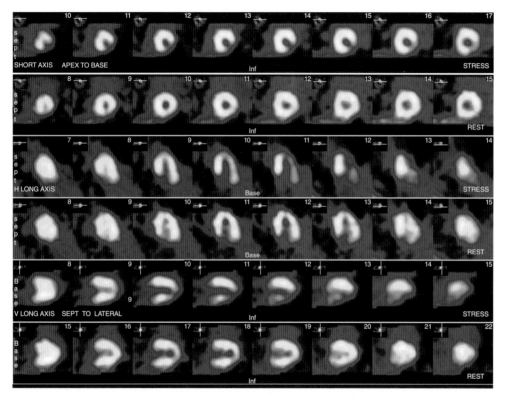

Figure 6.4 Stress and delayed (rest) SPECT myocardial perfusion images in the short-axis, vertical long-axis, and horizontal long-axis projections showing reversible perfusion scan defects consistent with a large area of inferolateral (left circumflex coronary artery) territory ischemia.

also be performed with a "first-pass" technique in which rapid serial imaging of the passage of a 99 m-Tc radiotracer bolus through the heart is used to calculate stress ventricular function. These techniques are infrequently used today as diagnostic tests for CAD.

Nuclear Perfusion Agents

Thallium-201 (^{201}Tl)

- ^{201}Tl is a metallic monovalent cation with biologic properties similar to potassium.
- Following intravenous (IV) injection, ^{201}Tl is rapidly extracted from the blood by the myocardium.
- Relatively little ^{201}Tl uptake by abdominal organs occurs during exercise. Therefore, interference with myocardial imaging by activity in the abdomen is relatively minor.
- The physical half-life of ^{201}Tl is 73 hours, which is practical for shipment and storage and allows for repeat imaging over time.
- ^{201}Tl decays to mercury-201, emitting mercury rays with energy of 69–83 keV (90%) and thallium gamma rays of 167 keV (10%). These emitted energies are at the low end of the energy range for gamma camera resolution; however they are acceptable for clinical use and allow adequate imaging with commercially available cameras.
- The usual IV dose of ^{201}Tl used for perfusion imaging is 3.5 millicuries (mCi). This ^{201}Tl dose results in an effective dose of 22 mSv. The effective dose is the weighted whole-body radiation dose used to compare different tests. The estimated yearly background effective dose is 3 mSv.
- Myocardial uptake of ^{201}Tl is dependent upon an active Na^+-K^+ ATPase pump, the intracellular concentration of ^{201}Tl achieved, the extraction fraction of isotope by the myocardium, and the distribution of regional myocardial blood flow.

- Only viable myocardial cells can take up (extract) and concentrate ^{201}Tl.
- The extraction fraction of ^{201}Tl by the myocardium is $88 \pm 2\%$ in resting dogs and is unaffected when heart rates HRs up to 195 beats per minute are induced with atrial pacing.
- At extremely low coronary blood flow rates, the extraction fraction of ^{201}Tl may be increased and thus overestimate blood flow.
- At maximal coronary flow rates induced by coronary vasodilator agents, the myocardial uptake of ^{201}Tl increases less than coronary blood flow.
- For practical purposes, over the physiologic range, ^{201}Tl distribution is proportional to regional blood flow and varies with it in a linear fashion.
- Myocardial ^{201}Tl activity reaches 80% of peak activity at one minute following injection. Peak myocardial activity occurs at 24 minutes following injection.
- As myocardial blood flow is progressively reduced (as in patients with CAD and flow-limiting stenoses) the percentage of peak activity reached in one minute is reduced and the time to peak myocardial ^{201}Tl activity is prolonged.
- Following initial myocardial extraction of ^{201}Tl, the subsequent concentration of isotope in the myocardium is determined by an equilibrium process between the blood pool and myocardial ^{201}Tl concentration.
- ^{201}Tl distribution after initial extraction by the heart is related to the balance between continued uptake of isotope into the myocardium from the blood pool and net ^{201}Tl washout from the myocardium (redistribution).
- ^{201}Tl uptake into myocardial territories supplied by coronary arteries without flow-limiting stenoses follows the kinetic profile described above. In hypoperfused myocardial regions supplied by coronary arteries with flow-limiting stenoses, ^{201}Tl uptake increases and peaks later as compared to normally perfused territories.
- As ^{201}Tl enters the myocardium under conditions of hyperemia following exercise or pharmacological-induced vasodilatation, the concentration of ^{201}Tl in the myocardium is significantly greater than that found in the blood pool. Therefore, the gradient driving ^{201}Tl from the myocardium into the blood pool is high and "washout" occurs over time.

- In hypoperfused areas of myocardium, the driving gradient between the myocardium and the blood pool is smaller and therefore the washout rate is significantly less. This phenomenon explains delayed ^{201}Tl redistribution.
- In clinical practice, areas of myocardium with uniform tracer uptake following exercise that show no significant quantitative difference in ^{201}Tl activity between exercise and rest are considered to represent normally perfused segments (Figure 6.2).
- Myocardial regions which demonstrate increased activity at rest as compared to the immediate post-stress images are considered to represent areas perfused by a significant, flow-limiting stenosis (Figures 6.3 and 6.4).
- A "fixed defect," in which diminished activity compared to other myocardial regions persists between stress and delayed (three to four hours post-stress) imaging, was formerly considered to represent irreversibly infarcted (scarred) myocardium. However, up to 49% of "fixed" defects on three- to four-hour delayed imaging may actually contain viable (ischemic) myocardium if additional delayed images and/or re-injection of additional ^{201}Tl (1–2 mCi) is performed.

Technetium-99m Sestamibi and Tetrofosmin

- Following IV injection, myocardial uptake of these ^{99m}Tc-labeled radiotracers is proportional to regional myocardial blood flow.
- The initial myocardial uptake of ^{99m}Tc-sestamibi and tetrofosmin depend upon an intact cell membrane and functioning mitochondria for uptake.
- After initial extraction, these ^{99m}Tc-labeled tracers localize in the mitochondria.
- The first-pass myocardial extraction fraction of ^{99m}Tc-sestamibi is only 40%. Within five minutes of injection, greater than 90% of isotope activity is cleared from the blood.

- A standard rest/stress study with 10/27.5 mCi of ^{99m}Tc-sestamibi results in a 11.3 mSv effective dose.
- As opposed to ^{201}Tl, clinical redistribution of ^{99m}Tc-sestamibi and tetrofosmin is minimal. The fractional clearance of ^{99m}Tc-sestamibi is ≤15% over a four-hour period from both areas with normal and reduced perfusion.

Advantages

^{99m}Tc-sestamibi and tetrofosmin possess certain advantageous physical characteristics which may make them more favorable as perfusion agents compared to ^{201}Tl:

- The peak emitted energy of 140 keV of ^{99m}Tc is at an ideal level for imaging with a gamma camera.
- Because of its higher energy, ^{99m}Tc is less attenuated by soft tissue than is ^{201}Tl. Therefore, images with ^{99m}Tc sestamibi and tetrofosmin are sharper and of better quality than with ^{201}Tl; a ^{99m}Tc-agent is considered a better isotope for imaging patients with larger amounts of soft tissue.
- The half-life of ^{99m}Tc is 6 hours, significantly shorter than that of ^{201}Tl (73 hours). This permits the use of ^{99m}Tc sestamibi or tetrofosmin doses 5–10 times higher than is feasible with ^{201}Tl.
- ^{201}Tl must be produced by a cyclotron and must be ordered in advance from the manufacturer. While many stress laboratories also order ^{99m}Tc sestamibi or tetrofosmin from outside radiopharmacies, these tracers also can be immediately produced by in-house generation. They are therefore more readily available for short-term and emergency use.
- Since minimal redistribution of ^{99m}Tc sestamibi occurs, it can be injected in the emergency department in patients during chest pain who can then undergo later imaging in the nuclear stress laboratory.
- As compared to ^{201}Tl where the timing of image acquisition is crucially important, the timing of ^{99m}Tc sestamibi or tetrofosmin image acquisition is less crucial thus allowing more flexible scheduling of image acquisition.
- Because of high count density, gated imaging with ^{99m}Tc-sestamibi and tetrofosmin is of higher quality than gated 201-Tl imaging. A first-pass left ventricular (LV) EF and assessment of regional wall motion (gated SPECT) can also be obtained.

Disadvantages

Certain disadvantages of ^{99m}Tc sestamibi and tetrofosmin are also recognized.

- Extensive hepatobiliary uptake relative to myocardial uptake is noted within the first hour following injection. Therefore, initial imaging after stress must be delayed for approximately one hour so that improved myocardial (in comparison to biliary) activity can be achieved. One hour after injection, approximately 6% of the injected dose is localized to the liver and 1% is concentrated in the heart.
- Due to the minimal redistribution noted with ^{99m}Tc sestamibi and tetrofosmin, separate rest and stress injections are required.

Stress Test and Radiotracer Protocols

- Each of the three clinically available perfusion agents has been administered to patients receiving standard exercise ECG treadmill testing or pharmacological stress testing.
- Patients should fast for three hours prior to the stress test to minimize gastrointestinal uptake of the perfusion agent.
- An indwelling IV catheter should be placed prior to the stress test.
- For patients undergoing treadmill exercise, the perfusion agent is administered at peak exercise and the patient is instructed to exercise at the peak level attained for an additional 45–60 seconds.
- Among patients undergoing vasodilator stress testing, the nuclear perfusion agent is administered at the time of peak coronary vasodilatation.
  - *Dipyridamole.* When dipyridamole is used for pharmacological vasodilator stress, a 0.56 mg/kg dose of dipyridamole is infused over four minutes: the myocardial perfusion agent is administered seven minutes after the start of the dipyridamole infusion.

- *Adenosine.* With adenosine infusion, the perfusion agent is injected during the adenosine infusion (administered at a dose of 140 mcg/kg/min). If a six-minute adenosine infusion is used, the tracer is injected at three minutes.
- *Regadenoson.* When using regadenoson, the vasodilator (0.4 mg dose) is injected over 10 seconds and is immediately followed by a 5 ml saline flush. The myocardial perfusion agent is then injected 10–20 seconds after the saline flush.
- Administration of aminophylline IV to reverse the stress vasodilator should be delayed for at least one minute (preferably two to three minutes) following injection of the nuclear perfusion agent so that coronary vasodilatation remains maximal during myocardial tracer extraction.
- *Dobutamine.* For patients receiving dobutamine infusion, the nuclear perfusion agent should be administered at peak dobutamine dose. Beta-blockers and/or nitrates should be held if at all possible for at least one minute following isotope injection.

^{201}Thallium

- At the peak of stress as described above, 3.5 mCi of ^{201}Tl is administered intravenously. Stress is continued for an additional 45–60 seconds to allow for maximal myocardial uptake of tracer.
- Due to ^{201}Tl redistribution, myocardial imaging should begin within 8–10 minutes following isotope injection in order to maximize detection of myocardial ischemia.
- SPECT images are obtained according to the protocols outlined above. In female patients with large breasts, the left breast should be shifted away from a position overlying the heart.
- Delayed (redistribution) images are obtained three to four hours later using the same technique to acquire the stress images, thus identifying areas of thallium redistribution and minimizing artifact.

- Food intake should be minimized between initial and delayed thallium imaging. Eating reduces blood thallium levels and diminishes thallium redistribution into ischemic myocardium.
- Patients with severe persistent (fixed) ^{201}Tl perfusion defects on delayed imaging may undergo re-injection with an additional 1 mCi of ^{201}Tl and have follow-up imaging to identify areas of potentially viable (hibernating) myocardium.
- Quantitative analysis software is typically used for image analysis along with visual assessment.

^{99m}Tc-sestamibi and Tetrofosmin

- Single-day imaging protocols with these tracers (usually rest preceding stress imaging) are currently used in most medical centers. Patients with marked obesity may undergo separate "2-day" imaging protocols.
- To perform rest imaging, 8–12 mCi of 99 m Tc-sestamibi or tetrofosmin is injected IV and imaging is performed approximately one hour later.
- At a later session, an exercise or pharmacological stress test is performed. At peak stress, 24–36 mCi of isotope is injected IV, and imaging is performed 45–60 minutes later, usually with a gated imaging acquisition protocol.
- Quantitative analysis software is typically used for image analysis along with visual assessment.

Combined ^{201}Tl and 99m Tc-sestamibi Protocol

- By taking advantage of the differing physical properties and kinetics of ^{201}Tl and 99 m Tc-sestamibi, selected centers may perform separate-acquisition dual isotope myocardial imaging to in order to compress the amount of time needed to perform a perfusion stress-rest acquisition.
- 3.0–3.5 mCi ^{201}Tl are administered IV at rest and images are collected 10 minutes later.

- Within 30 minutes following rest imaging, exercise or pharmacological stress is performed with injection of 20–30 mCi of 99m Tc-sestamibi or tetrofosmin at peak stress. Post-stress images are acquired 60 minutes later.
- A benefit of this protocol is the ability to perform 24-hour delayed ^{201}Tl imaging to assess the reversibility of fixed defects (identify viable myocardium).
- The disadvantage of this protocol is a high radiation dose of 29.2 mSv; use of this protocol is discouraged and it should only be used following the ALARA principle.

Image Interpretation

Nuclear Myocardial Perfusion Agents

- The interpretation of ^{201}Tl and 99m-Tc myocardial perfusion images is very similar. In order to optimally interpret myocardial perfusion images, the reader must appreciate variants of normal and commonly occurring imaging artifacts which if not recognized can lead to a false positive diagnosis of myocardial ischemia with poor diagnostic specificity.
- The multiple planar projection images (raw data) are reviewed for normal variants including:
  - Reduced activity at the base of the LV due to the presence of the aortic and mitral valves.
  - Decreased activity of the cardiac apex ("apical thinning") reflecting decreased myocardial thickness in this area.
  - Patient motion artifact.
  - "Upward creep" related to hyperventilation among patients with high exercise workloads, causing artifactual septal and inferior perfusion defects.
  - Technical artifacts such as non-uniformity in gamma camera detectors, center of rotation errors, misaligned cameras on multidetector scanner systems, and errors in image reconstruction.

- – Anterolateral and septal defects due to overlying breast tissue in women.
- – A high left hemidiaphragm which may attenuate activity at the posterobasal segment and the inferior wall.
- – Isolated septal perfusion defect in patients with left bundle branch block (LBBB).
- For purposes of image interpretation, myocardial segments are designated to correspond to the customary perfusion territory of a coronary artery.
  - – Anterior, anterolateral, and septal areas correspond to the distribution of the left anterior descending coronary artery.
  - – Inferior segments correspond to the right coronary artery distribution.
  - – Inferolateral and lateral segments correspond to the perfusion territory of the left circumflex coronary artery.
  - – The apical area most typically receives the majority of its blood supply from the left anterior descending artery, however significant contributions can emanate from the other coronary arteries, even in the same patient. Therefore, an isolated apical perfusion defect cannot be definitely assigned to the territory of a single coronary artery.
  - – A perfusion defect should be present in two or more projections on SPECT imaging to be considered indicative of ischemia.
- Normal myocardial perfusion is defined as homogeneous and full radiotracer distribution among all segments on both the resting and post-exercise scans (Figure 6.2).
- Reversible myocardial ischemia is present when a perfusion defect occurs on the post-stress scan and, in comparison, the resting scan shows improved or full radiotracer uptake in that segment (Figures 6.3 and 6.4).
- Perfusion defects may show partial or incomplete redistribution. This most frequently represents a combination of scar with surrounding ischemic myocardium as may be found following non Q-wave myocardial infarction or after reperfusion of a Q-wave myocardial infarction.
- Fixed defects are those which are present on the post-stress scan and which fail to improve (redistribute) on the resting scan. Fixed defects represent infarcted or scarred myocardium. In general, the severity of the perfusion

defect correlates with the viability of that myocardial segment. Fixed defects which are mild-to-moderate in severity usually represent partial infarct with residual viable myocardium. Moderate to severe fixed defects usually represent irreversibly scarred (infarcted) myocardium.

- As outlined above, re-injection of ^{201}Tl with repeated myocardial imaging may show evidence of perfusion (viability) in up to 49% of defects considered to be "fixed" after standard rest/redistribution imaging.
- Perfusion imaging with Tc-99m sestamibi after administration of nitroglycerin also may be useful for detection of viable myocardium.
- Multi-vessel CAD is suggested by reversible perfusion defects in more than one vascular supply territory.
- Other nuclear MPI scan findings indicative of severe CAD and adverse prognosis include:
  – Multiple transient perfusion defects in more than one vascular territory.
  – Increased lung uptake of isotope (after ^{201}Tl perfusion imaging) which reflects stress-induced LV dysfunction.
  – Transient post-stress LV cavity dilatation (increased stress-to-rest LV cavity ratio).
  – Diffuse, slow myocardial washout of ^{201}Tl with quantitative analysis suggesting multi-vessel or left main CAD.
  – Rest and/or post-stress left ventricular ejection fraction (LVEF) $\leq 45\%$.
  – Extensive ischemia/defects (involving >20% of the myocardium)
  – Large fixed defects.

Clinical Application of Nuclear Myocardial Imaging

Myocardial Perfusion Imaging

- MPI is indicated in patients with suspected CAD with a negative or non-diagnostic exercise ECG stress test and in those undergoing pharmacological stress testing.

- The sensitivity of SPECT imaging exceeds 80–90%. However, the reported specificity is lower because of technical factors, imaging artifacts, suboptimal count density, and referral bias. The "normalcy rate" (the proportion of patients with a very low pretest likelihood of CAD that had negative tests) exceeds 85–90%, however.
- MPI is useful in risk stratification of patients in whom exercise ECG stress testing suggests moderate risk, such as with an intermediate-risk Duke treadmill score (DTS).
- Gated SPECT imaging with 99m Tc-sestamibi or tetrofosmin, by allowing assessment of regional wall motion and myocardial thickening, may aid in recognition of tissue attenuation artifact (especially that involving the inferior wall with diaphragm or intestinal tissue), thereby improving the diagnostic accuracy of SPECT imaging.
- The reported sensitivity of exercise perfusion imaging increases as more vascular territories subtended by coronary arteries with significant stenoses are present. The sensitivity of MPI for single, double, and triple vessel CAD is 76, 86, and 90% respectively.
- In addition, the sensitivity for detection of CAD is higher in vascular territories supplied by vessels with ≥90% stenoses as opposed to those areas supplied by vessels with stenoses between 50 and 89%.
- Stress MPI provides enhanced diagnostic and prognostic information beyond that obtained from the exercise ECG test. The number and extent of transient (reversible) defects, lung uptake of radiotracer, and transient LV cavity dilatation with stress are important and significant independent predictors of future cardiac events.
- A completely normal myocardial perfusion scan predicts a low risk of future cardiac events (less than 1% annual risk) even in the presence of significant CAD documented by angiography. Stress MPI can therefore be employed to assess the efficacy of medical or revascularization therapy.
- Perfusion imaging can assess the hemodynamic (functional) significance of lesions detected by coronary angiography so that appropriate therapy (medical versus revascularization) can be prescribed.

Summary

- Nuclear myocardial imaging techniques are indicated in patients with pre-existing ECG abnormalities affecting repolarization, in those with an anticipated false positive or false negative ECG stress test, in those with equivocal, nondiagnostic, or intermediate-risk exercise ECG stress tests, and in those undergoing pharmacological stress testing.
- 99 m-Tc compounds are the predominant agents used in clinical practice, with Tl-201 used less commonly today.
- Nuclear imaging techniques improve the sensitivity, specificity, and diagnostic accuracy of the exercise ECG stress test.
- As opposed to the exercise ECG test, MPI allows better localization of ischemia to the vascular territories of the three major epicardial coronary arteries.
- SPECT imaging permits assessment of individual coronary supply territories. Gated SPECT imaging can determine LV volumes and EF.
- Nuclear imaging techniques provide important prognostic information beyond that available from the exercise stress ECG and hemodynamic response to exercise.
- Patients with a normal perfusion study have a very low risk (<1%/yr) of cardiac death or MI.
- Patients with reversible perfusion defects in multiple vascular territories, transient LV cavity dilatation, increased post-stress lung uptake of radiotracer, reduced LVEF, and increased LV volumes are at high risk of future cardiac events.
- To optimize sensitivity and specificity of MPI studies, identification of normal variants and imaging artifacts by an experienced reader is of paramount importance.
- Important differences in physical properties and kinetics exist among the clinically available nuclear perfusion agents. These differences necessitate variations in imaging protocols. In specific clinical situations a particular agent may be more suited for use than the others (examples: myocardial viability, ^{201}Tl more validated than 99 m Tc-agents; obesity, 99 m Tc-agents).

References

Depuey, E.G., Mahmarian, J.J., Miller, T.D. et al. (2012). Patient-centered imaging. *J. Nucl. Cardiol.* 19: 185–215. Erratum in: J Nucl Cardiol 2012; 19: 633. PMID: 22328324.

Dorbala, S., Ananthasubramaniam, K., Armstrong, I.S. et al. (2018). Single photon emission computed tomography (SPECT) myocardial perfusion imaging guidelines: instrumentation, acquisition, processing, and interpretation. *J. Nucl. Cardiol.* 25: 1784–1846.

Einstein, A.J., Moser, K.W., Thompson, R.C. et al. (2007). Radiation dose to patients from cardiac diagnostic imaging. *Circulation* 116: 1290–1305.

Fihn, S.D., Gardin, J.M., Abrams, J. et al., American College of Cardiology Foundation; American Heart Association Task Force on Practice Guidelines; American College of Physicians; American Association for Thoracic Surgery; Preventive Cardiovascular Nurses Association; Society for Cardiovascular Angiography and Interventions; Society of Thoracic Surgeons (2012). 2012 ACCF/AHA/ACP/AATS/PCNA/SCAI/STS guideline for the diagnosis and management of patients with stable ischemic heart disease: a report of the American College of Cardiology Foundation/American Heart Association task force on practice guidelines, and the American College of Physicians, American Association for Thoracic Surgery, Preventive Cardiovascular Nurses Association, Society for Cardiovascular Angiography and Interventions, and Society of Thoracic Surgeons. *J. Am. Coll. Cardiol.* 60: e44–e164.

Hachamovitch, R., Berman, D.S., Shaw, L.J. et al. (1998). Incremental prognostic value of myocardial perfusion single photon emission computed tomography for the prediction of cardiac death: differential stratification for risk of cardiac death and myocardial infarction. *Circulation* 97: 535–543.

Hendel, R.C., Berman, D.S., Di Carli, M.F. et al., American College of Cardiology Foundation Appropriate Use Criteria Task Force; American Society of Nuclear Cardiology; American College of Radiology; American Heart Association; American Society of Echocardiology; Society of Cardiovascular Computed Tomography; Society for Cardiovascular

Magnetic Resonance; Society of Nuclear Medicine (2009). ACCF/ASNC/ACR/AHA/ASE/SCCT/SCMR/SNM 2009 appropriate use criteria for cardiac radionuclide imaging: a report of the American College of Cardiology Foundation Appropriate Use Criteria Task Force, the American Society of Nuclear Cardiology, the American College of Radiology, the American Heart Association, the American Society of Echocardiography, the Society of Cardiovascular Computed Tomography, the Society for Cardiovascular Magnetic Resonance, and the Society of Nuclear Medicine. *J. Am. Coll. Cardiol.* 53: 2201–2229.

Henzlova, M.J., Duvall, W.L., Einstein, A.J. et al. (2016). ASNC imaging guidelines for SPECT nuclear cardiology procedures: stress, protocols, and tracers. *J. Nucl. Cardiol.* 23: 606–639.

7 Stress Echocardiography

Dennis A. Tighe

Introduction

Stress echocardiography is a robust and well-validated clinical method most frequently used for non-invasive evaluation of known or suspected coronary artery disease (CAD). A stress echocardiogram can be performed using either exercise stress (treadmill or bicycle ergometer) or pharmacological agents (dobutamine and vasodilators). The endpoint of stress echocardiography for detection of myocardial ischemia is development of stress-related hypoperfusion which manifests as a new or worsening regional wall motion abnormality (lack of wall thickening in association with stress-induced hypokinesia, akinesia, or dyskinesia) in a perfusion area subtended by a stenosed coronary artery. The technique has been shown to provide diagnostic and prognostic information comparable to that of radionuclide myocardial perfusion imaging (MPI). Stress echocardiography's advantages over MPI include its relatively lower cost, utility to identify other (potentially occult) cardiac pathologies, lack of patient exposure to ionizing radiation, and immediate availability of the results.

Pocket Guide to Stress Testing, Second Edition. Edited by Dennis A. Tighe and Bryon A. Gentile.
© 2020 John Wiley & Sons Ltd. Published 2020 by John Wiley & Sons Ltd.

As the markers of myocardial ischemia typically appear in a well-defined temporal cascade – the earliest alterations being flow heterogeneity between the subendocardial and subepicardial layers and metabolic changes, which are followed in sequence by the detectable clinical marker regional dysynergy, then ECG changes, global ventricular dysfunction, and finally chest pain – stress echocardiography offers the potential to diagnose CAD at an earlier stage and define the ischemic threshold.

In recent years, stress echocardiography has seen an expanded clinical role as the technique has become an established method for the assessment of a variety other cardiac conditions including the assessment of myocardial viability, native valvular heart disease, cardiomyopathies, diastolic heart failure, and prosthetic heart valves. This chapter reviews the various methods and applications of stress echocardiography.

Exercise Stress Echocardiography

Indications for Stress Echocardiography

The following are indications for exercise stress echocardiography:

- Detection of CAD when the resting ECG is abnormal or when a false positive or false negative result of exercise ECG testing is anticipated.
- Detection of CAD following a non-diagnostic exercise ECG test.
- Further assessment of an intermediate-risk Duke treadmill score (DTS) on standard exercise ECG stress testing.
- Evaluation for myocardial ischemia after a recent acute coronary syndrome (ACS) without revascularization or with incomplete revascularization.
- Assessment of mitral valve disease, including mitral regurgitation and mitral stenosis.

- Evaluation of patients with hypertrophic cardiomyopathy for assessment of left ventricle (LV) outflow tract gradients, mitral regurgitation, and pulmonary hypertension.
- Evaluation of dyspnea of possible cardiac origin.
- Assessment of patients following heart valve procedures where a discrepancy exists between symptom status and prosthetic valve hemodynamics.

Methods of Exercise Echocardiography

Bicycle Exercise Echocardiography

- Supine or upright bicycle ergometry techniques can be used to provide myocardial stress.
- A potential advantage of supine bicycle ergometry, compared to treadmill exercise or upright bicycle testing, is the ability to perform echocardiographic imaging during the stress bout. Given this capability, potential advantages of this technique include identification of the ischemic threshold and assessment of hemodynamic parameters (such as pulmonary artery systolic pressure and transvalvular and LV outflow tract pressure gradients) by Doppler echocardiography during the stress bout.
- The disadvantage of imaging during exercise is difficulty in obtaining high-quality images.
- Bicycle protocols, which are less used often in the United States, are highly dependent upon patient cooperation to maintain an adequate workload as compared to treadmill exercise.
- With cycle ergometry, the peak exercise work-load is about 10–20% lower compared to treadmill exercise.

Treadmill Exercise Echocardiography

- Treadmill exercise (see Chapter 5) is the most widely utilized method to perform exercise stress testing in the United States. Our laboratory almost exclusively uses treadmill testing for evaluation of CAD.

- With treadmill exercise, imaging is performed prior to stress and within one minute immediately following exercise without a "recovery period."

Examination Technique

Equipment
Exercise echocardiography requires the following equipment:

- Two-dimensional and Doppler echocardiographic system.
- Treadmill or bicycle ergometer.
- Continuous 12-lead ECG monitoring system.
- Blood pressure (BP) monitoring device.
- Imaging bed.
- Resuscitation equipment and medications.

Laboratory Layout
The physical layout of the room requires close proximity of the treadmill/upright bicycle to the echocardiograph and the imaging bed. The equipment placement is crucial because post-exercise imaging must be performed as rapidly as possible (within one minute) to maximize diagnostic yield.

Personnel
Required personnel include the qualified healthcare professional supervising the test, the echocardiographic technician, and (in some but not all laboratories) the stress ECG technician.

Preparations

- Patients are kept nothing per oral (NPO) for three hours prior to the test.
- Decisions about which medications to continue up to the time of the test should be made by the referring physician.
- After screening for appropriate indications and contraindications of exercise ECG testing (see Chapters 3 and 4), a standard resting 12-lead ECG is obtained.
- The patient should be oriented to the physical layout of the equipment and instructed to assume the left lateral decubitus position on the imaging bed immediately upon cessation of exercise.

Resting Stage

- Optimal pre-exercise echocardiographic images using harmonic imaging that maximize the definition of the LV endocardial border should be obtained in the parasternal short-axis, apical four-chamber, apical two-chamber, and apical three-chamber views (Figure 7.1). These images are recorded in cine-loop format so that side-by-side comparison to the post-exercise images can be made.
- When the endocardial definition is suboptimal, microbubble ultrasound contrast agents are indicated to enhance endocardial border definition; specifically when two or more LV segments are not well visualized. Intravenous access is required to administer one of these agents. Contrast agents can also be helpful in augmenting Doppler signals when hemodynamic assessments are made during stress echocardiography. Following protocols that optimize contrast administration will minimize the occurrence of technical issues such as under-filling of the LV and attenuation artifacts. Contrast echocardiography is not currently approved by the Food and Drug Administration (FDA) to assess myocardial perfusion.

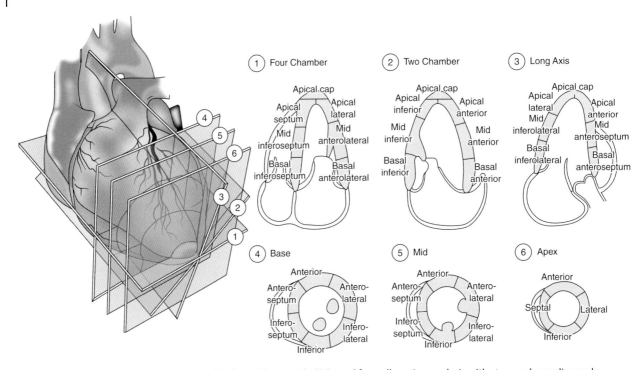

Figure 7.1 Diagram of the 17-segment model of the left ventricle (LV) used for wall motion analysis with stress echocardiography. *Source:* reproduced with permission from: Lang et al. (2005).

- The optimal transducer position used to acquire these images is marked on the chest wall to hasten the acquisition of the post-exercise images. The chest ECG leads must be appropriately placed so as not to interfere with these transducer positions.
- In addition to obtaining the images of LV used for analysis of wall motion, a baseline resting echocardiogram should be obtained prior to stress testing to include a screening assessment of biventricular function, chamber sizes, wall thicknesses, aortic root diameter, valvular structure and function, and presence of pericardial effusion. This imaging permits recognition of cardiac pathology that may be contributing to symptoms.

Exercise Phase

- Any standard graded exercise protocol can be used (see Chapter 5) for stress. In our laboratory, the Bruce protocol is most often used. Patients are encouraged to perform the maximum degree of exercise possible (symptom-limited) with a target heart rate (HR) set at 85% of age-predicted maximal HR.
- Continuous ECG monitoring is performed throughout the exercise period and vital signs are obtained during each stage of exercise. A 12-lead ECG should be acquired near the end of each stage.

Post-exercise Phase

- On completion of exercise, the patient is quickly stopped on the treadmill or upright bicycle and immediately returned to the imaging bed so that the post-exercise images can be expeditiously obtained. Patients undergoing supine bicycle stress need only turn into the left lateral decubitus position for imaging.
- Images for each of the views obtained in the pre-exercise stage are again acquired and recorded to a digitized cine-loop format. The resting and post-exercise images can then be compared in side-by-side fashion.

Interpretation of Exercise Stress Echocardiogram

- Supplementing the information derived from the ECG portion of the exercise test (symptoms, achieved workload, hemodynamic changes, ST-segment response, HR response, presence of arrhythmia), echocardiography provides an assessment of global and regional functional response to exercise.

Echocardiography Anatomy

- For adequate image interpretation, communication of results and correlation with other imaging modalities, the LV is divided into 16 or 17 anatomic segments (Figure 7.1).
- Although significant variability in the coronary artery blood supply to myocardial segments is known to exist, it is recommended that these segments be referred to the anticipated vascular supply distribution of the individual coronary arteries (Figure 7.2) to predict the location and extent of CAD:
  - Anteroseptal, anterior, anterolateral, and all apical segments correspond to the distribution of the left anterior descending coronary artery.
  - Inferoseptal and inferior segments correspond to the distribution of the right coronary artery.
  - Inferolateral segments correspond to the distribution of the left circumflex coronary artery.

Stress Responses (see Table 7.1)

- The normal response to progressive exercise is an increase in myocardial contractility and wall thickening in all segments, the LV cavity size becomes smaller, and the ejection fraction (EF) increases.
- A normal result of stress echocardiography is defined as normal LV wall motion at rest and with stress along with a decrease in LV cavity size and an increase in EF.

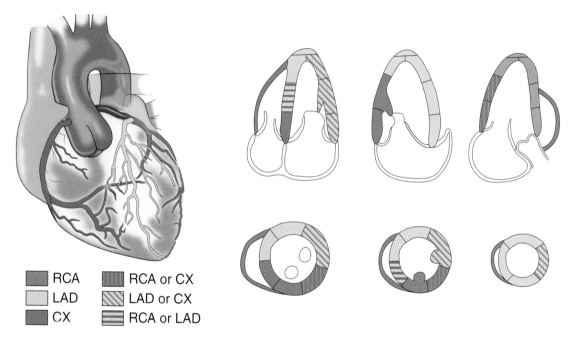

Figure 7.2 Diagram of regional wall segments and corresponding typical distribution of coronary artery perfusion territories. CX, left circumflex coronary artery; LAD, left anterior descending coronary artery; RCA; right coronary artery. *Source:* reproduced with permission from: Lang et al. (2015).

- An abnormal result of stress echocardiography is defined as any of the following responses to stress:
  - Development of a new wall motion abnormality compared to the rest study and/or failure of a segment to become hypercontractile (augment) with an adequate exercise workload; these responses should be considered indicators of myocardial ischemia.
  - A wall motion abnormality present on the rest study without change after exercise (fixed) is generally considered to represent myocardial scar (non-ischemic response). However, in some cases a fixed wall motion abnormality, especially if myocardial thickness is preserved, may represent myocardium perfused by a very severe stenosis (hibernating myocardium).
  - The occurrence of stress-induced LV cavity dilatation, failure of the LVEF to increase ≥5 EF points, and/or development of a new wall motion abnormality in more than one recognized vascular territory may indicate the presence of multi-vessel CAD.
  - While the primary focus of stress echocardiography should be on the imaging of the LV, a new wall motion abnormality or enlargement affecting the right ventricle has prognostic implications.
- Table 7.1 summarizes the interpretation of the imaging responses to stress echocardiography.

Accuracy of Exercise Stress Echocardiography

- Experienced, high-volume centers report that stress echocardiography is a highly accurate tool for detection of CAD. However, it is recognized that a steep "learning curve" exists for accurate interpretation of studies. Various quantitative means of analysis have been investigated, but the standard practice of interpretation of stress echocardiography remains visual assessment of LV wall motion and thickening; a method subject to inter-observer and inter-institutional variability.
- The sensitivities and specificities of exercise echocardiography for detection of CAD are reported to be 80–90% and 75–87%, respectively. When compared to exercise radionuclide MPI, exercise echocardiography exhibits a higher specificity and a somewhat lower sensitivity.

Table 7.1 Interpretation of responses to stress echocardiography.

Nature of tissue	Resting function	Low dose	Peak/post-stress function
Normal	Normal	Normal	Hyperkinetic
Ischemic	Normal	Normal (may worsen with severe CAD)	Worse than rest
Viable, ischemic	WMA at rest	Improvement	Reduction compared to low dose
Viable, non-ischemic	WMA at rest	Improvement	Sustained improvement
Infarction (scar)	WMA at rest	No change	No change

Source: Adapted with permission from: Marwick (2003).
CAD, coronary artery disease; WMA, wall motion abnormality.

- Sensitivity of the test is highest among patients with multi-vessel disease, and when the stenosis by angiography exceeds 70% of vessel diameter.
- Conversely, sensitivity is lower among those with single-vessel disease and when lesion severity is 50–70%.
- False negative studies are more common when an inadequate exercise workload is achieved (<85% predicted maximal HR, rate-pressure product <20 000), with use of anti-anginal medications, with poor LV endocardial definition, in the presence of concentric LV remodeling, delayed start (>1 minute) of post-exercise imaging and with single-vessel or circumflex CAD.
- False positive studies are more likely to occur when in the presence of pre-existing non-ischemic wall motion abnormality (such as with various cardiomyopathies), with poor LV endocardial definition, in the setting of left bundle branch block (LBBB), over-assessment of isolated basal inferior wall motion abnormality, and with a hypertensive response to stress.

Prognostic Value of Exercise Stress Echocardiography

Stress echocardiography has been shown to offer incremental benefit to clinical, resting echocardiography and exercise data. The presence and extent of inducible wall motion abnormalities on stress echocardiography can identify patients at increased risk of future cardiac events.

- In several studies, the annual cardiac event rate has been shown to increase as a function of the severity and extent of abnormal wall motion response during stress.
- A normal baseline and stress echocardiogram identifies a low annual risk (0.4–0.9%) for cardiac events in the subsequent four to five years, similar to that of normal stress MPI. This "warranty period" for a negative test does not necessarily appear to apply to patients with conditions such as chronic kidney disease and diabetes mellitus.
- Stress-induced wall motion abnormalities confer adverse risk for cardiac events; peak wall motion score index can risk stratify patients into low- (0.9%/year), intermediate- (3.1%/year), and high-risk (5.2%/year) groups for cardiac events.
- Transient ischemic dilatation of the LV cavity with stress has been shown to be a marker of severe and extensive angiographic CAD and is associated with a high risk of cardiac events.
- It is important to recognize that patients who achieve a submaximal age-predicted maximal HR in the setting of normal stress echocardiogram have a higher risk of cardiovascular events than those who attained a maximal level of stress.
- Similar to findings on exercise MPI, patients who are able to achieve high exercise workloads (≥10 metabolic equivalents [METs]) during testing often do not exhibit extensive wall motion abnormalities on stress imaging. In this setting, stress echocardiography does not appear to provide incremental prognostic information.

Dobutamine Stress Echocardiography

Pharmacology of Dobutamine

- Dobutamine is a short-acting, synthetic, catecholamine-like agent that directly acts as a stimulant of cardiac beta-receptors.
- Dobutamine was developed for use primarily as a positive inotropic agent (β-1 agonist) to augment cardiac contractility in patients with congestive heart failure (CHF); it has lesser chronotropic (β-2 agonist) and peripheral vascular (α-1 agonist) effects than other available catecholamine-like agents.
- The plasma half-life of dobutamine is two minutes, thus necessitating constant IV infusion to achieve the desired clinical effects.
- Substantially higher doses of dobutamine are required to perform stress echocardiography than are used therapeutically to treat CHF.
- In animal and human studies, a positive inotropic effect of dobutamine is observed prior to a significant chronotropic response.
- Dobutamine is estimated to increase coronary blood flow by approximately threefold over the level at rest.
- The increment in systolic BP produced by dobutamine is less when compared with exercise stress, thus rate-pressure products are lower with dobutamine infusion than with exercise stress. At higher dobutamine doses, a small decrease in BP may be observed due to activation of the β-2 adrenergic receptors and a vasodilatory effect.
- In myocardial segments subtended by an artery with a hemodynamically significant stenosis, the increase in myocardial oxygen demand created by the increased contractility and HR that accompany dobutamine infusion cannot be met with an appropriate increase in regional blood flow. Myocardial ischemia, manifested by a regional or segmental wall motion abnormality and lack of wall thickening, can be detected by echocardiography.

Indications for Dobutamine Stress Echocardiography

The following are indications for dobutamine stress echocardiography:

- Evaluation of known or suspected CAD among patients for who exercise ECG testing is inadequate.
- Evaluation of known or suspected CAD among patients for who stress testing with a vasodilator agent is contraindicated (see Chapter 8).
- Identification of myocardial viability among patients with suspected chronic ischemic LV dysfunction (hibernating myocardium).
- Risk stratification prior to non-cardiac surgery.
- Evaluation for myocardial ischemia after a recent ACS without revascularization or with incomplete revascularization.
- Assessment of patients with suspected low-flow, low-gradient aortic stenosis (defined as mean gradient <40 mmHg and aortic valve area <1.0 cm^2) with reduced LVEF (<50%) and low stroke volume (SV) index (<35 ml/m^2).
- Assessing contractile reserve among patients with dilated non-ischemic cardiomyopathies and among candidates for cardiac resynchronization therapy.
- Assessment of patients following heart valve procedures where a discrepancy exists between symptom status and prosthetic valve hemodynamics.

Patients with LBBB on ECG can be assessed using dobutamine stress echocardiography, but in our experience evaluation with a vasodilator-MPI test is the preferred method.

Contraindications of Dobutamine Stress Echocardiography

The infusion of dobutamine is contraindicated with the following conditions:

- Active unstable angina pectoris.
- Acute myocardial infarction (MI) within one to three days.

- Complex, uncontrolled ventricular ectopy.
- Uncontrolled atrial tachyarrhythmia.
- Hypertrophic obstructive cardiomyopathy.
- Aortic dissection.
- Moderate to severe systemic hypertension (resting systolic blood pressure (SBP) >180 mmHg).
- Known hypersensitivity reaction to dobutamine.
- Large or symptomatic aortic aneurysm (relative contraindication).

Examination Technique

Equipment

The required equipment for dobutamine stress echocardiography includes:

- Two-dimensional and Doppler echocardiographic system.
- Continuous 12-lead ECG monitoring system.
- BP monitoring device.
- Infusion pump to deliver dobutamine.
- Imaging bed.
- Atropine, IV beta-blocker, nitrates.
- Resuscitation equipment and medications.

Personnel

The required personnel for dobutamine stress echocardiography include the supervising qualified healthcare professional, echocardiographic technician, and, in some but not all laboratories, a stress ECG technician.

Patient Preparation

- Patients are kept NPO for three hours prior to testing.
- Beta-blockers can blunt the inotropic and chronotropic effects of dobutamine; however, supplemental atropine can be administered to overcome the HR-limiting effects of beta-blockers. Oftentimes, beta-blockers are held prior to testing. The decision on continuation of beta-blocker therapy should depend on the clinical objectives of the test.
- After screening for appropriate indications and contraindications, a standard resting 12-lead ECG is obtained and examined.

Resting Stage

- The baseline (resting) echocardiographic images are obtained in the apical four-chamber, apical two-chamber, apical long-axis, and parasternal short-axis views. The images are recorded in the digital cine-loop format so side-by-side comparison of these images can be made with those obtained during the various stages of infusion.
- When the endocardial definition is suboptimal, microbubble ultrasound contrast agents should be used to enhance endocardial border definition.
- As for exercise stress echocardiography, a screening baseline echocardiogram should be obtained to identify any potential cardiac pathology that may be contributing to symptoms.
- If the resting images are technically adequate for evaluation of the LV endocardium, an 18 or 20 gauge IV catheter is placed in an arm vein for infusion of dobutamine and other medications.

Infusion Stage

- In our laboratory, we currently use a pre-mixed solution of dobutamine at a concentration of 2 mg/ml for infusion. This solution is then run through an infusion pump system to purge any air bubbles which may be present.
- Other medications which should be immediately available include:
  - Atropine sulfate 2 mg for IV administration.
  - An intravenous β-blocker (metoprolol, esmolol).
  - Nitroglycerin for sublingual use.
  - Phentolamine mesylate to minimize tissue injury should extravasation of dobutamine occur.

Administration

- Dobutamine infusion is initiated at either a dose of 2.5, 5, or 10 mcg/kg/min depending upon various institutional protocols and goals of the test.
- For assessment of suspected or known CAD, the most common indication for dobutamine stress echocardiography, we initiate the dobutamine infusion at 10 mcg/kg/min (some institutions begin the protocol at 5 mcg/kg/min).
  - At three-minute intervals, the infusion rate is increased by increments of 10 mcg/kg/min until a maximum infusion rate of 40 mcg/kg/min is achieved.
  - If an established endpoint does not occur, atropine is administered IV in 0.5 mg aliquots every 30–60 seconds to a maximum of 2.0 mg in order to achieve the target HR and increase the sensitivity of the test, particularly in patients receiving β-blockers and those with milder CAD.
  - Alternative methods to achieve target HR include performing a sustained, firm hand grip on a soft rubber ball, a technique shown to raise BP as well as HR (used in our laboratory when required), continuing the 40 mcg/kg/min dose for a total of five minutes (minimizes the use of atropine and its attendant risk of faster HR and increased risk of side effects), or increasing the infused dose of dobutamine up to 50 mcg/kg/min (not routinely performed in our laboratory).

- For the evaluation of hibernating myocardium, our protocol begins at an infusion rate of 2.5 mcg/kg/min for five minutes, then proceeds to a 5 mcg/kg/min infusion for five minutes, and then to 10 mcg/kg/min for an additional five minutes. Most segments that are "viable" will show augmentation at these low infusion rates and display reduced contractility at higher infused doses ("biphasic response"). If infusion of dobutamine to higher rates is required to assess for myocardial ischemia, the protocol described above is then followed.
- For the assessment of conditions not related to evaluation of myocardial ischemia, the peak infused doses of dobutamine generally should not exceed 10–20 mcg/kg/min. A growing indication in stress laboratories is referral for evaluation of patients with low-flow, low-gradient aortic stenosis with reduced LVEF. Our protocol for this indication follows the recommendations of the European Association of Cardiovascular Imaging and the American Society of Echocardiography (Table 7.2).
- Continuous ECG monitoring for analysis of rhythm and ST-segment response is performed during infusion and the recovery phase until the HR has returned to the baseline level.
- A 12-lead ECG and BP measurement are obtained at the end of each infusion stage.
- Digitized images from low-dose (5 or 10 mcg/kg/min), peak dose, and recovery phase are saved in continuous cine-loop format and compared to the resting (pre-infusion) images.

Endpoints

The endpoints for termination of dobutamine infusion include:

- Achievement of pre-determined target HR (85% age-predicted maximal HR for all protocols except among those experiencing a recent ACS in whom 70% of predicted maximal HR is used).
- Development of a new segmental wall motion abnormality.
- Development of significant ventricular or atrial arrhythmias.
- Ischemic chest pain.

Table 7.2 Low-dose dobutamine protocol for suspected low-flow, low-gradient aortic stenosis.

Starting dobutamine dose of 2.5–5 mcg/kg/min

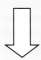 Increase dose 2.5–5 mcg/kg/min every 3–5 minutes

Maximum dobutamine dose of 20 mcg/kg/min

Infusion stopped when:
- Maximum dobutamine dose reached (20 mcg/kg/min).
- Positive result obtained.
- Heart rate rises 10–20 bpm over baseline or exceeds 100 bpm.
- Symptoms, blood pressure fall, or significant arrhythmias.

Positive results defined as:
- Increase in effective valve area to >1.0 cm^2; suggests that stenosis is not severe.
- Severe stenosis is suggested by a jet velocity >4.0 m/sec or mean gradient >30–40 mmHg provided that the valve area does not exceed 1.0 cm^2 at any flow rate.
- Lack of contractile reserve (failure to increase stroke volume [SV] >20%).

Source: Adapted with permission from: Baumgartner et al. (2017).

- ECG changes suggesting severe myocardial ischemia.
- Development of severe hypertension (SBP ≥220 mmHg and/or diastolic blood pressure (DBP) ≥120 mmHg).
- Development of significant hypotension (≥20 mmHg decline of SBP with symptoms).
- Patient request due to side effects.
- Completion of protocol.

Complications of Dobutamine Stress Echocardiography

- Side effects are more frequent with higher infused doses of dobutamine and when supplemental atropine is used.
- Non-cardiac side effects occur in about 25% of patients. The most frequent side effects include nausea, anxiety, headache, tremor, and urinary urgency.
  - Non-cardiac side effects rarely (≤3% of tests) require test termination.
- Cardiac side effects are more frequent. Chest pain typical of angina occurs in 20% of patients, ST-segment depression of ≥1 mm in 10%, hypotension (variable definitions) in about 14–37% (≥20 mmHg in 20% and as a test endpoint in 1.7%), and severe hypertension in 1.3%.
- The mechanism of hypotension during dobutamine infusion is debated. Some investigators believe that enhanced inotropic state with dynamic intra-cavitary and LV outflow tract obstruction is causative. Other investigators postulate that a vasodepressor response to dobutamine is partially responsible. A third explanation depends upon the definition of "hypotension" and the observation that a significant association exists between higher resting SBP and hypotension during dobutamine infusion.
- Arrhythmia is the most common cardiac side effect encountered, occurring in approximately 30% of patients receiving dobutamine and atropine.
- The most frequent arrhythmias encountered are ventricular premature contractions (15%), atrial premature contractions (7.8%), and supraventricular tachycardia (1.3%). Atrial fibrillation or flutter rarely occurs (<1%) with dobutamine infusion.

- Non-sustained ventricular tachycardia (VT) occurs in 0.2–4% of patients.
  - Most arrhythmias are transient and self-limiting; specific treatment is seldom needed.
- Life-threatening complications, including death (<0.01%), MI (0.02%), ventricular fibrillation (0.04%) and sustained VT (0.15%), are rare.

Interpretation of Dobutamine Stress Echocardiography (see Table 7.1)

- Similar to exercise echocardiography, a 16- or 17-segment model of the LV is used (Figure 7.1).
  - The normal response to progressive dobutamine infusion is development of hyperdynamic wall motion and enhanced myocardial thickening in all segments and a reduction in LV cavity size.
  - The development of a new regional wall motion abnormality compared to the resting study and/or the failure of a segment to become hypercontractile with progressive dobutamine infusion are indicators of myocardial ischemia.
  - A resting wall motion abnormality without change from resting after dobutamine infusion is generally considered to represent myocardial scar, but in some cases may represent a myocardial region supplied by a vessel with a very severe stenosis (hibernating myocardium).
  - Resting akinesis which becomes dyskinesis with stress usually reflects a purely passive, mechanical consequence of increased intraventricular pressure developed by normally contracting walls and should not be considered indicative of active ischemia.
  - Dobutamine-induced LV cavity dilatation and hypokinesis in more than one recognized vascular territory is a highly specific indicator of multi-vessel CAD.
  - The observation of a "biphasic response," increased contractility at low dose (2.5–5.0 mcg/kg/min) dobutamine infusion and subsequent "redevelopment" of a wall motion abnormality when higher doses (>10 mcg/kg/min) are infused, is a highly specific indicator of hibernating and potentially viable myocardium.
- Table 7.1 summarizes the interpretation of the imaging responses to dobutamine stress echocardiography.

Sensitivity and Specificity

- The reported sensitivity of dobutamine stress echocardiography is approximately 85–90%; the reported specificity is 80–85%.
- Sensitivity is higher with more extensive CAD and when lesion severity exceeds 90% diameter stenosis.
- Factors which may contribute to false negative tests include inadequate myocardial stress, use of β-blockers, inadequate echocardiographic imaging, and vigorous contractility with enhanced wall motion at higher infused dobutamine doses.
- False positive studies are most frequent among patients with resting wall motion abnormalities, such as with cardiomyopathy, LBBB, or mitral valve prolapse.
- The development of a new regional wall motion abnormality at a HR ≤125 bpm is associated with a higher likelihood of multi-vessel disease than when ischemia is detected at a higher HR.
- ST-segment depression occurring with dobutamine infusion is reported to have poor sensitivity and limited specificity for detection of CAD.
- Unlike the significance of hypotension that occurs during exercise ECG testing, hypotension during dobutamine infusion is not associated with advanced CAD or adverse prognosis.
- Bradycardia during dobutamine infusion is not a marker of CAD.
- In comparison to nuclear perfusion imaging, dobutamine stress echocardiography exhibits similar sensitivity and higher specificity.

Advantages of Dobutamine Stress Echocardiography

The advantages of dobutamine echocardiography over nuclear MPI include:

- Ability of echocardiography to identify other cardiac pathologies (cardiomyopathy, valvular heart disease, left ventricular hypertrophy (LVH), pericardial disease, pulmonary hypertension, unsuspected wall motion abnormalities).

- Higher specificity.
- Overall lower cost.
- More rapid test performance and reporting of results.
- Greater convenience for the patient.
- Ability to define an "ischemic threshold".
- Lack of patient exposure to ionizing radiation.

Disadvantages of Dobutamine Stress Echocardiography

The general disadvantages of dobutamine-atropine stress echocardiography include:

- As compared to exercise stress echocardiography, dobutamine echocardiography is time-intensive, because dobutamine infusion may require more than 20 minutes for an endpoint to be reached and the post-procedure recovery period may be prolonged when high-dose dobutamine and supplemental atropine are used.
- At high infused doses of dobutamine, excessive cardiac motion may occur, which can obscure wall motion abnormalities, and lead to a false negative test result.
- Side effects are frequent with high infused dobutamine dosage and when atropine is required.
- Lower reported sensitivity compared to testing with vasodilator-MPI.

Other Methods of Stress Echocardiography

- Stress echocardiography can be performed using other pharmacologic agents and methodologies.
- Infusion of dipyridamole (0.84 mg/kg over 10 minutes) has been the most widely studied stress agent, although adenosine (140 mcg/kg/min over six minutes) has been used in conjunction with echocardiography. In comparison

with vasodilator agents (dipyridamole and adenosine), dobutamine has higher sensitivity, generally better tolerated side effects, and is a superior agent to assess for wall motion abnormalities. Vasodilator stress echocardiography is seldom used in the United States, but its use is more common in Europe.

- Transesophageal dobutamine stress echocardiography has been reported to be a safe, feasible, and accurate technique to detect CAD among patients with inadequate transthoracic echocardiographic windows.
- When a permanent pacemaker is in place, its presence can be exploited to perform a pacing stress test by externally programming the pacemaker to gradually increase the HR.
- Transesophageal atrial pacing in conjunction with transthoracic or transesophageal echocardiography has also been described as a highly sensitive and specific technique for detecting CAD in selected patients.

Summary

- Stress echocardiography is a mature and robust clinical method for the diagnosis of CAD and assessment of prognosis. In recent years, several non-coronary indications for stress echocardiography have emerged.
- Stress echocardiography can be accomplished with exercise stress or the use of pharmacological agents. Dobutamine is the most widely used pharmacological agent used for stress echocardiography in the United States.
- The diagnostic accuracy of stress echocardiography is equivalent to that achieved with the use of myocardial perfusion agents. In general, stress echocardiography is more specific, but less sensitive than MPI.
- Stress echocardiography is limited among patients who have poor transthoracic echocardiographic images. Microbubble (ultrasonic enhancing) contrast agents should be used for LV opacification when indicated to improve test performance.
- A 16-or 17-segment model of the LV is used for interpretation of the stress echocardiogram.

- The normal response to progressive stress is increased contractility and wall thickening in all myocardial segments and a reduction in LV cavity size.
- A new wall motion abnormality compared to rest and/or failure of a segment to become hypercontractile with stress is indicative of myocardial ischemia.
- Advantages of stress echocardiography over MPI include lower cost, more rapid availability of results, higher specificity, patient convenience, ability to identify an ischemic threshold, portability of echocardiography, ability to identify other cardiac pathologies with baseline echocardiography, and lack of ionizing radiation exposure.
- Disadvantages of stress echocardiography include limited echocardiographic windows in up to 10–15% of patients, the steep learning curve required to adequately perform and interpret tests, potential for prolonged test duration with dobutamine infusion, and lower sensitivity compared to MPI.

References

Bangalore, S., Yao, S., and Chaudhry, F.A. (2007). Role of right ventricular wall motion abnormalities in risk stratification and prognosis of patients referred for stress echocardiography. *J. Am. Coll. Cardiol.* 50: 1981–1989.

Baumgartner, H., Hung, J., Bermejo, J. et al. (2017). Recommendations on the echocardiographic assessment of aortic valve stenosis: a focused update from the European Association of Cardiovascular Imaging and the American Society of Echocardiography. *J. Am. Soc. Echocardiogr.* 30: 372–392.

Cerqueira, M.D., Weissman, N.J., Dilsizian, V. et al., American Heart Association Writing Group on Myocardial Segmentation and Registration for Cardiac Imaging (2002). Standardized myocardial segmentation and nomenclature for tomographic imaging of the heart. A statement for healthcare professionals from the Cardiac Imaging Committee of the Council on Clinical Cardiology of the American Heart Association. *Circulation* 105: 539–542.

Fleischmann, K., Hunink, M., Kuntz, K., and Douglas, P. (1998). Exercise echocardiography or exercise SPECT imaging? A meta-analysis of diagnostic test performance. *JAMA* 280: 913–920.

Geleijnse, M.L., Krenning, B.J., Nemes, A. et al. (2010). Incidence, pathophysiology, and treatment of complications during dobutamine-atropine stress echocardiography. *Circulation* 121: 1756–1767.

Heijenbrok-Kal, M.H., Fleischmann, K.E., and Hunink, M.G. (2007). Stress echocardiography, stress single-photon-emission computed tomography and electron beam computed tomography for the assessment of coronary artery disease: a meta-analysis of diagnostic performance. *Am. Heart J.* 154: 415–423.

Lancellotti, P., Pellikka, P.A., Budts, W. et al. (2017). The clinical use of stress echocardiography in non-ischaemic heart disease: recommendations from the European Association of Cardiovascular Imaging and the American Society of Echocardiography. *J. Am. Soc. Echocardiogr.* 30: 101–138.

Lang, R.M., Badano, L.P., Mor-Avi, V. et al. (2015). Recommendations for cardiac chamber quantification by echocardiography in adults: an update from the American Society of Echocardiography and the European Association of Cardiovascular Imaging. *J. Am. Soc. Echocardiogr.* 28: 1–39.

Lang, R.M., Bierig, M., Devereux, R.B. et al. (2005). Recommendations for chamber quantification: a report from the American Society of Echocardiography's Guidelines and Standards Committee and the Chamber Quantification Writing Group, developed in conjunction with the European Association of Echocardiography, a branch of the European Society of Cardiology. *J. Am. Soc. Echocardiogr.* 18: 1440–1463.

Marwick, T.H. (2003). Stress echocardiography. *Heart* 89: 113–118.

Pellikka, P.A., Nagueh, S.F., Elhendy, A.A. et al. (2007). American Society of Echocardiography recommendations for performance, interpretation, and application of stress echocardiography. *J. Am. Soc. Echocardiogr.* 20: 1021–1041.

Picano, E., Alaimo, A., Chubuchny, V. et al. (2002). Noninvasive pacemaker stress echocardiography for diagnosis of coronary artery disease: a multicenter study. *J. Am. Coll. Cardiol.* 40: 1305–1310.

Porter, T.R., Mulvagh, S.L., Abdelmoneim, S.S. et al. (2018). Clinical applications of ultrasonic enhancing agents in echocardiography: 2018 American Society of Echocardiography guidelines update. *J. Am. Soc. Echocardiogr.* 31: 241–274.

Wolk, M.J., Bailey, S.R., Doherty, J.U. et al., American College of Cardiology Foundation Appropriate Use Criteria Task Force (2014). ACCF/AHA/ASE/ASNC/HFSA/HRS/SCAI/SCCT/SCMR/STS 2013 multimodality appropriate use criteria for the detection and risk assessment of stable ischemic heart disease: a report of the American College of Cardiology Foundation Appropriate Use Criteria Task Force, American Heart Association, American Society of Echocardiography, American Society of Nuclear Cardiology, Heart Failure Society of America, Heart Rhythm Society, Society for Cardiovascular Angiography and Interventions, Society of Cardiovascular Computed Tomography, Society for Cardiovascular Magnetic Resonance, and Society of Thoracic Surgeons. *J. Am. Coll. Cardiol.* 63: 380–406.

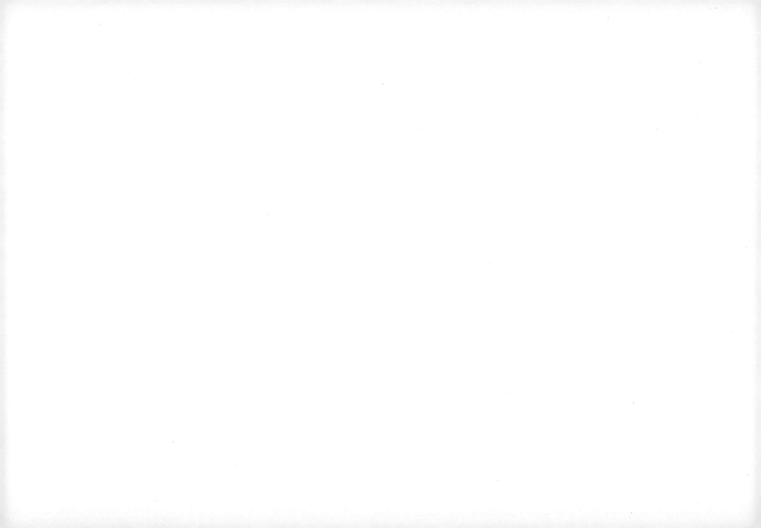

8 Pharmacological Stress Testing

Dennis A. Tighe

Introduction

Exercise ECG stress testing is the preferred method to evaluate for suspected coronary artery disease (CAD) and to assess functional status. However, certain patients cannot perform an adequate exercise test for a variety of reasons (Table 8.1). In this situation, the use of pharmacological agents, including vasodilators or beta-adrenergic stimulants, in conjunction with a myocardial imaging technique can be substituted for exercise ECG stress testing with equivalent results for detection and localization of ischemic myocardium. The hemodynamic response to exercise, however, cannot be reproduced with the available pharmacological agents. This chapter reviews the indications and use of pharmacological stress testing agents.

Pocket Guide to Stress Testing, Second Edition. Edited by Dennis A. Tighe and Bryon A. Gentile.
© 2020 John Wiley & Sons Ltd. Published 2020 by John Wiley & Sons Ltd.

Table 8.1 Indications for pharmacologic stress testing.

- Limiting orthopedic injury
- Musculoskeletal deformities
- Limiting neurologic deficit
- Limiting peripheral vascular disease
- Evaluation of coronary artery disease (CAD) with inadequate exercise ECG test workload
- Preoperative assessment of patients awaiting non-cardiac surgery
- Evaluation of CAD in patients with fixed left bundle branch block (LBBB) or ventricular pacing
- Risk assessment post uncomplicated acute coronary syndrome

Vasodilator Agents

Currently three coronary vasodilator agents are available for clinical use: dipyridamole, adenosine, and regadenoson. In recent years, regadenoson has become the preferred vasodilator agent used in many stress laboratories, however, both dipyridamole and adenosine find continued use.

Dipyridamole (Persantine®)

General Considerations

- Dipyridamole is a potent vasodilator agent, which acts by blocking the cellular uptake and transmembrane transport of endogenous adenosine and by inhibiting adenosine breakdown by the enzyme adenosine deaminase.

- The vasodilatory action of dipyridamole is not strictly limited to the coronary arterioles, however, as a less pronounced effect on the peripheral circulation is noted.
- Coronary blood flow in normal coronary arteries is increased four to fivefold above resting levels in response to dipyridamole infusion due to enhanced coronary vasodilatation (normal "flow reserve").
- In coronary arteries with a hemodynamically significant stenosis, the vascular bed distal to the narrowing is already dilated at rest (decreased vascular resistance/flow reserve) to a certain degree. Therefore, the vasodilator response to dipyridamole is attenuated and subendocardial flow is restricted.
- The resulting "flow heterogeneity" between vascular beds with normal and diminished flow reserve in response to vasodilator infusion can be detected with myocardial imaging techniques.
- "True myocardial ischemia" is less common, but can be induced by an increased rate-pressure product or more likely by a steal phenomenon between the subepicardium and subendocardium when the vasodilator flow reserve is exceeded.
- The hemodynamic effects associated with dipyridamole infusion include:
  - An approximate 20% increase in heart rate (HR) over baseline.
  - An approximate 10–15 mmHg fall in systolic blood pressure (SBP).
  - A small increase in rate-pressure product due to increased HR.
- The hemodynamic effects of dipyridamole are more pronounced among patients who develop ST-segment depression associated with dipyridamole infusion.
- ST-segment depression develops in 8–40% (average 10–12%) of patients undergoing dipyridamole stress testing. ST-segment depression is considered a highly specific, but insensitive marker of significant CAD.
- Dipyridamole-^{201}Tl scanning has been extensively studied and used for the preoperative evaluation of cardiac risk before vascular surgery.
- Due to the high incidence of false positive septal perfusion abnormalities associated with exercise perfusion imaging, vasodilator agents, such as dipyridamole, have found extensive use among patients with left bundle branch block (LBBB) and ventricular pacing for stress testing.

Contraindications

The following conditions are contraindications to dipyridamole use:

- Bronchospastic lung disease with ongoing wheezing or a history of significant reactive airway disease.
- SBP <90 mmHg.
- Uncontrolled hypertension (SBP >200 mmHg or diastolic blood pressure [DBP] >110 mmHg).
- Ingestion of caffeinated foods or beverages (e.g. coffee, tea, sodas) within the last 12 hours (Table 8.2).
- Unstable angina or less than two to four days after acute myocardial infarction (MI).
- Known hypersensitivity to dipyridamole.

Side Effects

- Adverse effects occur in 40–50% of patients who receive dipyridamole infusion. Most effects are self-limiting, and serious side effects are rare.
- Non-cardiac side effects such as headache, flushing, dizziness, and gastrointestinal upset are frequent.
- Chest pain occurs in 10–25% of patients receiving dipyridamole. It is an insensitive marker of significant CAD.
- Atrioventricular (AV) block occurs at a lower frequency than is observed with adenosine and regadenoson.
- Acute MI and cardiac death have rarely been associated with dipyridamole infusion.
- Acute bronchospasm is a serious side effect which requires immediate therapy. In this situation, the dipyridamole infusion should be immediately terminated, and IV aminophylline (75–250 mg) should be administered. Inhaled bronchodilators may be required.
- Acute neurologic events (stroke, transient ischemic attack) have been reported to occur in association with dipyridamole infusion. Patients with recent neurologic symptoms due to vascular insufficiency or evidence of severe cerebral vascular disease should not be considered candidates for dipyridamole stress testing.

Protocols for Administration

- Patients should fast for at least three hours before testing in order to minimize the risk of nausea and emesis and to diminish splanchnic blood flow so that radiotracer accumulation within the heart is maximized.
- Methylxanthine medications (Table 8.2) should be discontinued a minimum of 36–48 hours prior to the test because they limit the vasodilatory effect of dipyridamole, resulting in decreased diagnostic utility. For similar reasons, caffeine-containing medications and products (Table 8.2) should be withheld for 12–24 hours prior to testing.
- Concomitant myocardial imaging is required due to the low incidence of ST-segment shifts associated with the use of dipyridamole. Myocardial perfusion imaging (MPI) (see Chapter 6) is most often employed, however protocols for dipyridamole stress echocardiography are available.
  - An antecubital vein should be used in preference to a hand vein for IV access because smaller veins are more sensitive to the acidic pH of dipyridamole.
- The patient should be in the supine position at the time of dipyridamole infusion. Baseline (pre-infusion) ECG, HR, and blood pressure (BP) should be obtained and recorded.
- Continuous ECG monitoring is performed and vital signs are obtained every 2 minutes during infusion and for up to 10 minutes thereafter.
- The standard dose of dipyridamole for IV infusion is weight-based: 0.57 mg/kg over a period of four minutes (0.142 mg/kg/min)
- As the proper weight-based dose for obese patients is unclear, the maximum recommended dose is based on a weight of 250 pounds or 125 kg.
- Dipyridamole-induced hyperemia lasts for more than 50 minutes. Peak vasodilation after dipyridamole administration occurs on average 6.5 minutes after the start of the infusion. The half-life of dipyridamole is approximately 30–45 minutes.

Table 8.2 Methylxanthine derivatives and caffeine-containing products.

Methylxanthines
- Theophylline preparations (many brand names)
- Oxtriphylline preparations
- Aminophylline (theophylline ethylenediamine) preparations
- Dyphylline preparations
- Pentoxifylline

Caffeine-containing medications (common)
- Anacin products
- Bayer Back and Body
- Cafergot products
- Darvon compounds
- Excedrin products
- Fioricet
- Fiorinal products
- Goodys products: extra strength tablets, extra strength headache powder, cool orange powder
- Midol products
- No Doz products
- Vanquish analgesic tablets
- Vivarian
- Zantrex-3 weight-loss supplement

Caffeine-containing foods and beverages[a]
- Coffees
- Teas
- Cocoa
- Chocolate (candy, drinks, ice cream, and yogurt)
- Colas
- Sodas (non-colas): Mountain Dew, Mountain Zevia, Dr. Pepper, Sunkist Orange, Barq's Root Beer
- Energy drinks
- Ice creams and yogurt (coffee flavor, Bang caffeinated ice cream)
- Caffeinated snack foods

[a] A more complete list is available at: https://cspinet.org/eating-healthy/ingredients-of-concern/caffeine-chart (accessed December 15, 2018).

- The myocardial perfusion agent is injected three to five minutes after completion of the dipyridamole infusion (time of peak vasodilatory effect). The imaging protocol followed depends upon which radiotracer agent is used (see Chapter 6).
- Aminophylline (75–250 mg) can be given IV to reverse the coronary vasodilatory and adverse side effects of dipyridamole should the situation require it. At least one minute should elapse between injection of the MPI agent and administration of aminophylline to insure optimal imaging.
- For dipyridamole echocardiography, a dose of 0.84 mg/kg is administered IV over 10 minutes (0.56 mg/kg over 4 minutes, no drug for 4 minutes, and then 0.28 mg/kg over 2 minutes). Echocardiography is performed at rest and during the 10 minute infusion.

Clinical Results

- The reported sensitivity and specificity of dipyridamole myocardial perfusion imaging is 85 and 91% respectively. Sensitivity is higher among patients with multi-vessel as opposed to single vessel CAD.
- A normal dipyridamole myocardial perfusion imaging scan is associated with an excellent long-term cardiac event-free risk, however, the "warranty period" is less than that found for normal exercise MPI.
- The use of echocardiography in conjunction with dipyridamole is less reliable in many centers than is nuclear imaging for a diagnosis of myocardial ischemia because focal wall motion changes are less common with dipyridamole than are nuclear scan defects associated with flow heterogeneity.
- Dipyridamole infusion can be supplemented by the performance of exercise to increase the rate-pressure product in an attempt to increase diagnostic accuracy of the test and the image quality of the myocardial perfusion scan.
  - After infusion of dipyridamole, isometric handgrip can be performed for three to five minutes while the patient is in the supine position. Conflicting results regards to coronary blood flow augmentation and concentration of radiotracer within the myocardium noted in various studies limits the clinical applicability of supplemental isometric handgrip.

- Patients who are ambulatory may undergo low-level exercise (e.g. treadmill 1.7 mph, 0% grade) for four to six minutes just after the completion of the dipyridamole infusion. The myocardial perfusion imaging agent is injected during this low-level exercise, and the exercise is continued for an additional two minutes to allow for tracer uptake in the myocardium.
- Low-level treadmill exercise requires that the patient be upright, and it is more labor intensive than isometric handgrip. Among patients undergoing low-level exercise immediately following dipyridamole infusion, the incidence of non-cardiac side effects is lessened, the incidence of ST-segment depression is doubled, and myocardial concentration of radiotracer is improved as blood flow is diverted away from the splanchnic bed and to the heart.
- Low-level exercise supplementation is not recommended for patients with LBBB, Wolff-Parkinson-White (WPW), and ventricular pacing due to HR-related imaging artifacts.

Adenosine (Adenoscan®)

General Considerations

- Adenosine is an endogenous nucleoside with potent vasodilator effects that non-specifically activates several sub-types of adenosine receptors.
- The coronary vasodilatory effect of adenosine appears to be mediated through activation of the A2A receptor.
- Coronary blood flow increases four to sixfold over basal levels during adenosine infusion.
- The biologic half-life of adenosine is <10 seconds necessitating constant IV infusion. Therefore, its vasodilator effect and side effects are short-lived.
- Peak vasodilation after adenosine administration occurs within one to two minutes after the start of the infusion.
- The hemodynamic effects of adenosine parallel those associated with dipyridamole:
  - HR increases on average by 15 bpm.
  - Systolic and diastolic BPs are reduced by roughly 10%.
  - Rate-pressure product mildly increases.

Contraindications

Contraindications to adenosine infusion include the following:

- Bronchospastic lung disease with ongoing wheezing or a history of significant reactive airway disease.
- Second- or third-degree AV block without a functioning pacemaker in place.
- Sinus node disease, such as sick sinus syndrome or symptomatic bradycardia, without a functioning pacemaker in place.
- SBP <90 mmHg.
- Uncontrolled hypertension (SBP >200 mmHg or DBP >110 mmHg).
- Recent (<48 hours) use of dipyridamole or dipyridamole-containing medications.
- Unstable angina or less than two to four days after acute MI.
- Known hypersensitivity to adenosine.

Side Effects

- Side effects are more frequent with adenosine infusion (70–80% of patients) as compared to dipyridamole use. Side effects are related to activation of other adenosine receptor subtypes (A1, A2B, and A3 receptors).
- The most common side effects encountered include non-specific chest pain, dyspnea, and flushing due to activation of A2B receptors.
- An additional side effect encountered with adenosine that is rarely observed with dipyridamole is AV block, mediated by adenosine interaction with the A1 receptor.
  - First degree AV block occurs in 5–10% of patients.
  - Second degree AV block (usually Mobitz-type I) occurs in 4–5% of cases.
  - Advanced AV block occurs in ≤1% of patients.
- Most cases of AV block are self-limiting and rarely associated with significant hemodynamic effects. A decrease in the infusion rate or termination of adenosine infusion may be required in some cases.

- Induction of atrial fibrillation has been reported as a consequence of adenosine infusion.
- As opposed to dipyridamole, most side effects associated with adenosine infusion are transient in nature, due to the short half-life of adenosine. Most adverse effects respond promptly (within one to two minutes) to termination of the infusion. Administration of aminophylline is rarely required.
- ST-segment depression ≥1 mm occurs in 5–7% of patients receiving adenosine. This finding has high specificity for CAD.
- Acute bronchospasm is a serious adverse effect (mediated by adenosine interaction with the A2b and A3 receptors). Therapy includes immediate discontinuation of the adenosine infusion and prompt administration of IV aminophylline.

Protocol for Administration

- As with dipyridamole, patients should fast for ≥3 hours prior to the test.
- Methylxanthine medications should be withheld for 36–48 hours prior to testing.
- Caffeine-containing medications and products should be withheld 12–24 hours prior to the time of testing.
- Oral dipyridamole should also be held due to the risk of seriously potentiating adenosine-induced side effects (especially advanced AV block).
- Baseline 12-lead ECG, HR and BP are recorded. Two IV cannulas are inserted in large arm veins: one for infusion of adenosine and one for administration of the radiotracer agent. In some institutions, only one IV cannula is inserted and a three-way stopcock is placed in the infusion circuit necessitating brief interruption of adenosine infusion to inject the myocardial perfusion imaging agent.
- Continuous ECG monitoring is performed. Vital signs are recorded every minute during infusion.
- The standard weight-based dose of adenosine is 140 mcg/kg/min administered by continuous IV infusion for six minutes. The correct weight-based dose for obese patients is unclear. It is suggested that the maximum dose that should be based on a weight of 250 pounds (or 125 kg). An infusion pump is required.
- Because maximal coronary vasodilatation occurs within two to three minutes of commencing the adenosine infusion, the radiotracer is administered at three minutes and not post-infusion, as is the case with dipyridamole.

- In some laboratories, a shorter duration adenosine infusion protocol, lasting four minutes, has been used. For this shorter duration protocol, the minimum time to radiotracer injection should be two minutes, and the infusion should continue for at least two minutes after radiotracer injection.
- Patients who are ambulatory may undergo low-level exercise (e.g. treadmill 1.7 mph, 0% grade) during the adenosine infusion. This low-level exercise may decrease the frequency of adenosine-related side effects, attenuate the drop in BP associated with adenosine, and lead to improved image quality on the perfusion imaging scan. As with dipyridamole, low-level exercise supplementation is not recommended for patients with LBBB, WPW, and ventricular pacing due to HR-related imaging artifacts.
- In rare instances, the infused dose may be slowly titrated from 70 mcg/kg/min up to the full, recommended dose. Side effects may necessitate reduction of the infused dose or termination of infusion, if severe.
- Imaging protocols following radiotracer injection depend upon which agent is used (see Chapter 6).

Clinical Results

- The reported sensitivity and specificity of adenosine perfusion imaging for identifying CAD exceeds 80–90%. Sensitivity is highest among patients with multi-vessel disease.
- The sensitivity and specificity of adenosine echocardiography is less than that reported for adenosine MPI or dobutamine stress echocardiography.

Regadenoson (Lexiscan®)

General Considerations

- Regadenoson is a highly selective A2A adenosine receptor agonist which exhibits very low affinity for other endogenous adenosine receptors (A1, A2B, and A3).

- Activation of the A2A adenosine receptors by regadenoson produces coronary vasodilation and increases myocardial blood flow.
- Regadenoson has found great clinical utility because of its specific affinity for the A2A adenosine receptor which permits a maximal vasodilator effect with rapid termination of action (permitting bolus dosing) while limiting side effects that accompany activation of other adenosine receptor subtypes.
- With injection of regadenoson, peak hyperemia starts within 30 seconds and persists for 2–4 minutes.
- The hemodynamic effects due to regadenoson injection are similar to those of adenosine:
  - HR increases on average by 25 bpm (greater than with adenosine).
  - Systolic and diastolic BPs are reduced by about 10–15 mmHg.
  - Rate-pressure product mildly increases.

Contraindications

Contraindications to use of regadenoson for stress testing include the following:

- Bronchospastic lung disease with ongoing wheezing or a history of significant reactive airway disease.
- Second- or third-degree AV block without a functioning pacemaker in place.
- Sinus node disease, such as sick sinus syndrome or symptomatic bradycardia, without a functioning pacemaker in place.
- SBP <90 mmHg.
- Uncontrolled hypertension (SBP >200 mmHg or DBP >110 mmHg).
- Unstable angina or less than two to four days after an acute MI.
- Recent (<48 hours) use of dipyridamole or dipyridamole-containing medications.
- Known hypersensitivity to adenosine or regadenoson.

Side Effects

- Compared with adenosine, most of the side effects associated with regadenoson occur less commonly and appear to be better tolerated. Most of the side effects experienced with regadenoson are mild and transient in nature.
- The most common adverse reactions of regadenoson injection include shortness of breath (25–30%), headache (25%), chest pains (30%), and flushing (20%).
- Other side effects may include dizziness/lightheadedness (7%), gastro-intestinal discomfort (20–25%), throat/ neck/jaw pain (7%), and dysgeusia/metallic taste (5%).
- The majority of side effects occur soon after dosing and usually resolve within 15 minutes; an exception being headache, which may take up to 30 minutes to resolve.
- For severe and/or persistent adverse reactions, IV aminophylline (75–250 mg) may be administered at least two to three minutes after radiotracer injection.
  - Recently, Doran and colleagues showed that 60 mg of IV caffeine over three to five minutes can be an effective agent for reversal of regadenoson effects, equivalent to IV aminophylline. For mild symptoms, oral caffeine appears to a reasonable first choice, reserving IV aminophylline or IV caffeine for symptoms that do not resolve or when gastrointestinal or other symptoms preclude the ability to drink a caffeinated beverage.
- As compared to adenosine, AV block is less commonly encountered, consistent with the weak interaction of regadenoson with adenosine A1 receptor.
  - First-degree AV block occurs in 3% of patients.
  - Second-degree AV block occurs in 0.1% of patients.
- Most cases of AV block are self-limiting and rarely associated with significant hemodynamic effects.
- Cases of asystole and prolongation of the QT-interval have been reported.
- ST-segment depression occurs in about 12% of patients receiving regadenoson.
- New-onset or recurrent atrial fibrillation and atrial flutter have been reported following regadenoson administration.

- Some rare, but potentially serious adverse reactions related to regadenoson injection have been reported including:
  - New onset or recurrence of convulsive seizures.
  - Refractory myocardial ischemia and infarction.
  - Hemorrhagic and ischemic cerebrovascular accidents.

Protocol for Administration

- As with the other vasodilator agents used for stress testing, patients should fast for ≥3 hours prior to the test.
- Methylxanthine preparations should be withheld for 36–48 hours prior to testing.
- Caffeine-containing medications and products should be withheld at least 12 hours prior to the time of testing.
- Oral dipyridamole, or medications containing dipyridamole, should be withheld for at least 48 hours prior to regadenoson administration.
- A baseline ECG and HR and BP should be recorded. A single 22 gauge IV cannula should be inserted in an arm vein.
- Continuous ECG monitoring is performed. Vital signs are recorded.
- The recommended dose of regadenoson is 0.4 mg (5-ml solution) given as an IV injection within 10 seconds. A 5-ml saline solution flush should be administered immediately after the injection of regadenoson.
- The myocardial perfusion imaging radiotracer should be injected 10–20 seconds after the saline flush. The same IV line used for regadenoson may be used.
- Patients who are ambulatory may undergo low-level exercise (e.g. treadmill 1.7 mph, 0% grade for 1.5 minutes) followed by regadenoson injection and tracer injection followed by an additional 2 minutes of exercise. This low-level exercise leads to improved image quality on the perfusion imaging scan. As with the other vasodilator agents, low-level exercise supplementation is not recommended for patients with LBBB, WPW, and ventricular pacing due to HR-related imaging artifacts.

Clinical Results

- As compared to adenosine myocardial perfusion imaging, regadenoson induces equivalent scintigraphic results as adenosine regarding the size and severity of left ventricle (LV) perfusion defects and the extent of ischemia.
- The prognostic implications of normal and abnormal regadenoson-MPI are demonstrated to be similar to adenosine-MPI.

Beta-Adrenergic Agonist

Dobutamine

General Considerations

- Dobutamine is a synthetic catecholamine developed primarily to be a positive inotropic (β_1-agonist) agent with lesser effects on HR and BP than other available catecholamines.
- Dobutamine also has cardiac chronotropic (β_2-agonist) activity and is an α-adrenergic antagonist (vasodilator) on the peripheral vasculature.
- The plasma half-life of dobutamine is two minutes, therefore it must be administered by continuous IV infusion to achieve desired hemodynamic effects.
- Concomitant myocardial imaging is required with dobutamine infusion to identify ischemic or potentially viable myocardium.
- Dobutamine infusion is the preferred method of pharmacological stress testing among patients with reactive airways disease, those receiving theophylline preparations, and those with cerebrovascular disease.

- Among patients with resting LBBB or ventricular pacing, vasodilators are the preferred method of pharmacologic stress. If dobutamine is used in this situation, echocardiography appears to be the imaging modality of choice due to reported cases of false-positive septal radionuclide perfusion scan defects.
- The primary disadvantage of dobutamine stress testing is the possibility that a prolonged time period (exceeding 20 minutes) may be required to complete the infusion protocol and recovery phase.

Contraindications

The infusion of dobutamine is contraindicated with the following conditions:

- Active unstable angina pectoris.
- Acute MI (within one to three days).
- Complex, uncontrolled ventricular ectopy.
- Uncontrolled atrial tachyarrhythmia.
- Hypertrophic obstructive cardiomyopathy.
- Known hypersensitivity reaction to dobutamine.
- Aortic dissection.
- Moderate to severe systemic hypertension (resting SBP >180 mmHg or DBP >110 mmHg).
- Large or symptomatic aortic aneurysm (relative contraindication).

Side Effects

- The side effect profile of dobutamine is more favorable than that of the vasodilators. Comparisons of dipyridamole, adenosine and dobutamine in the same group of patients showed that dobutamine was better tolerated with the least number of side effects.

- Cardiac side effects of dobutamine include:
  - Chest pain in 15–20% of patients
  - Palpitation in 10–30%
  - Arrhythmia in 25–30%
  - Hypotension (variable clinical definitions) in 14–38%
- Most cardiac side effects are well tolerated and self-limited with discontinuation of dobutamine infusion. In some cases, the side effects can be more severe and may require administration of IV β-blockers or nitrates for ischemic complications, IV fluids for symptomatic hypotension, or antiarrhythmic drugs for sustained/symptomatic arrhythmia.
- ST-segment depression is infrequent (<10% of cases) and is a non-specific marker of CAD.
- Hypotension has many potential causes including vasodilatation, myocardial ischemia, volume depletion, arrhythmia, or dynamic LV outflow tract obstruction.
- Non-cardiac side effects include:
  - Nausea in 8% of patients
  - Anxiety in 6%
  - Headache in 4–9%
  - Tremor in 10%
  - Flushing in 14%
- As with cardiac side effects, most non-cardiac adverse reactions are well-tolerated and rarely require termination of the infusion.
- In general, side effects occur more frequently at higher infused doses of dobutamine and when supplemental atropine is administered.

Protocol for Administration
Preparations for the Test

- The patient should be fasting for at least three hours prior to the test.
- If possible, β-blockers should be held since they may blunt the inotropic and chronotropic response to dobutamine infusion.
- A baseline 12-lead ECG is obtained prior to testing, and an IV catheter is securely placed in an arm vein.
- Other medications which should be immediately available include:
  - Atropine sulfate 1–2 mg (contraindicated in patients with angle-closure glaucoma).
  - IV β-blocker (metoprolol, esmolol).
  - Nitroglycerin.
  - All other medications indicated for emergency cardiac care.
- Phentolamine mesylate, an α-adrenergic blocking agent, should also be available in the unusual event of tissue extravasation of dobutamine. If extravasation occurs, the dobutamine infusion should be immediately terminated, the IV cannula should be removed, and the affected extremity should be elevated. Then 5–10 mg of phentolamine diluted in 10 ml of 0.9% sodium chloride should be administered into the area with a fine needle.

Dobutamine Infusion

- At our institution, a pre-mixed solution of dobutamine at a concentration of 2 mg/ml is used.
- A programmable infusion pump is used to deliver dobutamine at the desired initial concentration and to facilitate rapid upward dose titration during the infusion protocol.
- Continuous ECG monitoring is performed throughout the test. The HR and BP are recorded at baseline and with each incremental stage of dobutamine infusion.

- Echocardiography is the imaging technique most often performed in conjunction with administration of dobutamine. Resting (baseline) two-dimensional images in the parasternal short-axis view and the apical four-, apical three-, and two-chamber views are acquired. Digitized images are saved to the echocardiograph in a continuous cine-loop quad screen format.
- When the endocardial definition is suboptimal, microbubble ultrasound contrast agents should be used to enhance endocardial border definition.
- Once adequate resting images are acquired, dobutamine infusion is initiated at a dose of 10 mcg/kg/min for three minutes and increased by 10 mcg/kg/min to a maximum dose of 40 mcg/kg/min (some laboratories use a maximum dose of 50 mcg/kg/min) or until another endpoint is achieved (Table 8.3).
- In some laboratories, the initial dose of dobutamine is 5 mcg/kg/min for three minutes with subsequent dose escalation as described above.

Table 8.3 Endpoints of dobutamine infusion.

- Development of a new segmental wall motion abnormality
- Significant atrial or ventricular arrhythmia
- Achievement of ≥85% age-predicted maximal heart rate (HR)
- Ischemic chest pain associated with ST-segment depression
- Severe hypertension
- Hypotension (systolic blood pressure [SBP] <90 mmHg)
- Other significant side effect(s)
- Patient requests to stop
- Completion of protocol

- Supplemental atropine in 0.5 mg aliquots to a total dose of 2.0 mg can be given IV if target HR has not been achieved and the patient is clinically stable.
- Digitized images in the views described above are also acquired at a low infused dobutamine dose (usually 10 or 20 mcg/kg/min), peak infused dose, and during recovery for comparison to baseline images.
- If myocardial viability is at issue, the infusion can be started at a low-dose (2.5 or 5 mcg/kg/min) using five-minute stages initially to assess for contractile reserve in myocardial segments which are severely hypokinetic at rest.
- When myocardial perfusion tomography is used as the imaging technique, dobutamine infusion is initiated and up-titrated as described above for stress echocardiography in order to achieve the target HR.
- The radiotracer should be injected at the time of peak HR as the dobutamine infusion is continued for an additional one minute. Stress and rest imaging is subsequently scheduled according to which particular radiotracer has been given (see Chapter 6).

Endpoints

- Standard endpoints for termination of infusion are followed (Table 8.3).
- If ≥85% maximal predicted HR has not been achieved, supplemental atropine can be given or exercises, such as isometric hand-grip or low-level foot exercises, can be performed.

Clinical Results (see Chapters 6 and 7)

- The normal response to progressive dobutamine infusion is augmentation of myocardial contractility and wall thickening in all segments and reduction in LV cavity size. The development of a new wall motion abnormality (hypokinesis, akinesis, or dyskinesis) and/or LV cavity dilatation represents an ischemic response and implies the presence of functionally significant CAD.
- Myocardial segments that are hypokinetic or akinetic at rest and that fail to augment with progressive dobutamine infusion are considered to represent infarcted tissue (scar).

- Worsening of a pre-existing wall motion abnormality during infusion represents myocardial ischemia.
- Hypokinetic or akinetic segments that augment at low dose (2.5–5 mcg/kg/min) and that subsequently fail to augment or develop worsening systolic function with progressive dobutamine infusion ("biphasic response") likely represent areas of viable myocardium.
- The sensitivity and specificity of dobutamine stress echocardiography for detection of angiographic CAD is 80 and 84% respectively. In comparison to dobutamine-MPI, the sensitivity is slightly lower, but specificity is higher; the overall diagnostic accuracy is similar.

Summary

- Exercise ECG testing (with or without myocardial imaging) is the preferred method to pharmacological stress to evaluate for suspected CAD when patient can perform an adequate exercise bout.
- Pharmacological stress testing is indicated when patients are unable to perform adequate exercise or when exercise ECG testing is inadequate (Table 8.1).
- Vasodilator agents and dobutamine can be used to provide myocardial stress. Table 8.4 summarizes the characteristics of the clinically available pharmacologic stress agents and Figure 8.1 illustrates time lines for their administration and associated nuclear MPI agent protocol.
- Concomitant myocardial imaging is required when pharmacological stress agents are used due to the low incidence of ST-segment alterations induced by these agents.
- Myocardial perfusion imaging is the preferred technique when vasodilator agents are used.
- Conversely, echocardiography is the preferred imaging technique for use with dobutamine infusion.
- The sensitivity and specificity of pharmacologic stress imaging to detect CAD is equivalent to that of exercise stress myocardial imaging.
- Vasodilator imaging is the preferred technique if fixed LBBB or ventricular pacing is present.
- Dobutamine is the preferred agent for patients with bronchospastic lung disease.

Table 8.4 Comparison of available pharmacologic stress agents.

	Dipyridamole	Adenosine	Regadenoson	Dobutamine
Mechanism of action	Vasodilator	Vasodilator	Vasodilator	Positive inotrope and chronotrope
Customary IV dose	0.57 mg/kg over 4 min for perfusion imaging 0.84 mg/kg over 10 min for echo	140 mcg/kg/min for 6 min	0.4 mg/5 ml IV injection over 10 seconds	5–40 mcg/kg/min
Contraindications	Bronchospastic lung disease, acute myocardial infarction (MI), unstable angina, symptomatic cerebral vascular disease	Bronchospastic lung disease, acute MI, unstable angina, symptomatic cerebral vascular disease, 2°/3° AV block	Bronchospastic lung disease, acute MI, unstable angina, symptomatic cerebral vascular disease, 2°/3° AV block	Acute MI, unstable angina, severe hypertension, uncontrolled arrhythmia, hypertrophic cardiomyopathy
Plasma half-life	10 hr	<10 sec	2–4 min (initial phase), 30 min (intermediate phase), 2 hr. (terminal phase)	2 min
Side effects	Frequent, can be long-lasting	Frequent, transient	Frequent, transient	Less frequent, mild, transient
Antidote	Aminophylline	Aminophylline	Aminophylline, Caffeine	β-blockers, nitrates
Elimination	Liver	Endothelium, erythrocytes	Renal	Liver
Preferred imaging strategy	Nuclear perfusion agents	Nuclear perfusion agents	Nuclear perfusion agents	Echocardiography
Special uses	LBBB, ventricular pacing, preoperative evaluation	LBBB, ventricular pacing, preoperative evaluation	LBBB, ventricular pacing, preoperative evaluation	Patients with bronchospastic lung disease, myocardial viability

Source: Adapted in part and with permission from: van Rugge et al. (1992) and Dilsizian et al. (2015).

(a) Dipyridamole-MPI imaging protocol

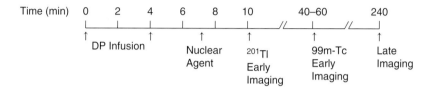

(b) Adenosine-MPI agent imaging protocol

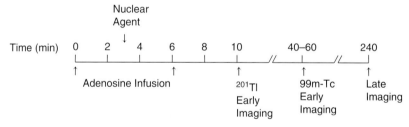

Figure 8.1 Time-line diagrams for pharmacological agent-myocardial perfusion imaging. Tc, technetium; Tl, thallium.

(c) Regadenoson-MPI agent imaging protocol

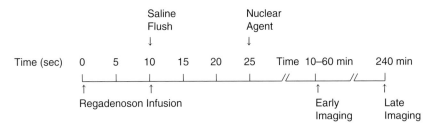

(d) Dobutamine-MPI agent imaging protocol

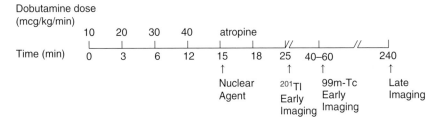

Figure 8.1 (Continued)

References

Al Jaroudi, W. and Iskandrian, A.E. (2009). Regadenoson: a new myocardial stress agent. *J. Am. Coll. Cardiol.* 54: 1123–1130. Erratum in: *J. Am. Coll. Cardiol.* 2009; 54: 1635.

Cerqueira, M.D., Verani, M.S., Schwaiger, M. et al. (1994). Safety profile of adenosine stress perfusion imaging: results from the Adenoscan Multicenter Trial Registry. *J. Am. Coll. Cardiol.* 23: 384–389.

Dilsizian, V., Gewirtz, H., Paivanas, N. et al. (2015). Serious and potentially life threatening complications of cardiac stress testing: physiological mechanisms and management strategies. *J. Nucl. Cardiol.* 22: 1198–1213.

Doran, J.A., Sajjad, W., Schneider, M.D. et al. (2017). Aminophylline and caffeine for reversal of adverse symptoms associated with regadenoson SPECT MPI. *J. Nucl. Cardiol.* 24: 1062–1070.

Farzaneh-Far, A., Shaw, L.K., Dunning, A. et al. (2015). Comparison of the prognostic value of regadenoson and adenosine myocardial perfusion imaging. *J. Nucl. Cardiol.* 22: 600–607.

Geleijnse, M.L., Elhendy, A., Fioretti, P.M., and Roelandt, J.R. (2000). Dobutamine stress myocardial perfusion imaging. *J. Am. Coll. Cardiol.* 36: 2017–2027.

Geleijnse, M.L., Fioretti, P.M., and Roelandt, J.R. (1997). Methodology, feasibility, safety and diagnostic accuracy of dobutamine stress echocardiography. *J. Am. Coll. Cardiol.* 30: 595–606.

Geleijnse, M.L., Krenning, B.J., Nemes, A. et al. (2010). Incidence, pathophysiology, and treatment of complications during dobutamine-atropine stress echocardiography. *Circulation* 121: 1756–1767.

Henzlova, M.J., Duvall, W.L., Einstein, A.J. et al. (2016). ASNC imaging guidelines for SPECT nuclear cardiology procedures: stress, protocols, and tracers. *J. Nucl. Cardiol.* 23: 606–639. Erratum in: *J. Nucl. Cardiol.* 2016; 23: 640–642.

Lette, J., Tatum, J.L., Fraser, S. et al. (1995). Safety of dipyridamole testing in 73,806 patients: the Multicenter Dipyridamole Safety Study. *J. Nucl. Cardiol.* 2: 3–17.

Mahmarian, J.J., Cerqueira, M.D., Iskandrian, A.E. et al. (2009). Regadenoson induces comparable left ventricular perfusion defects as adenosine: A quantitative analysis from the ADVANCE MPI 2 trial. *JACC Cardiovasc Imaging* 2: 959–968.

van Rugge, F.P., van der Wall, E.E., and Bruschke, A.V.G. (1992). New developments in pharmacologic stress imaging. *Am. Heart J.* 124: 481.

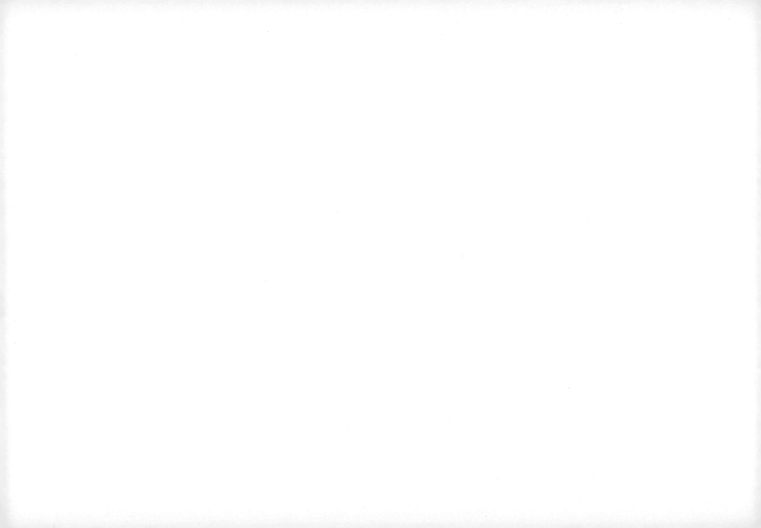

9 Cardiopulmonary Exercise Testing

Bryon A. Gentile

Introduction

Aerobic exercise capacity is an important predictor of adverse events across a wide spectrum of patient populations. A recent meta-analysis reported a 13% decrease in all-cause mortality and 15% decrease in cardiovascular events for each 1-MET (metabolic equivalent) increase in maximal aerobic capacity (MAC).

As a result, exercise testing remains one of the most widely utilized non-invasive assessments in patients with cardiovascular disease due to its diagnostic and prognostic value. As with any other diagnostic test, it has been refined, over time, to include echocardiographic and nuclear imaging techniques and more recently with incorporation of ventilatory expired gas analysis. The combination of exercise testing and gas exchange analysis is commonly referred to as cardiopulmonary exercise (CPX) testing, and provides the most accurate assessment of MAC.

This chapter will provide a basic review of CPX testing, including its clinical applications, with a focus on the use in patients with heart failure (HF) and unexplained dyspnea.

Physiology

Aerobic exercise represents a balance between the cardiovascular and respiratory systems' ability to supply oxygen in exchange for carbon dioxide to meet the metabolic needs of working muscles and organs. This complex process can be simplified into four categories:

- Pulmonary ventilation: the movement of oxygenated air into and deoxygenated air out of the lungs.
- Pulmonary diffusion: the exchange of oxygen and carbon dioxide between the alveoli and capillaries of the lungs.
- Transportation of oxygenated blood to the muscles and organs.
- Capillary diffusion: the exchange of oxygen and carbon dioxide between capillaries and muscle.

During exercise, the respiratory and cardiovascular systems must augment ventilation, diffusion, and transportation to meet the metabolic demands of increased workloads.

Pulmonary Adaptations to Exercise

To meet the metabolic demands of the body during exercise, the respiratory system must increase oxygen supply. This is accomplished by a proportional increase in minute ventilation ($\dot{V}_E$), through increases in respiratory rate and tidal volume.

Tidal volume represents the volume of air displaced with normal respiration. A fraction of this volume reaches the alveoli where gas is exchanged, the remainder occupies what is referred to as dead space (V_D).

Although dead space volume increases during exercise, due to dilation of the bronchial tree, the overall tidal volume also increases, resulting in an increase in alveolar ventilation.

Cardiovascular Adaptations to Exercise

Expected cardiovascular responses to exercise are reviewed in Chapters 14 and 19. Briefly, the increased myocardial oxygen demand of muscle is met by an increase in cardiac output (Q), which may increase by as much as sixfold during exercise. Cardiac output is augmented by an increase in heart rate (HR) (chronotropy) and stroke volume (SV) (inotropy), as well as distribution away from the splanchnic bed.

Pulmonary and peripheral vasodilation allows for greater oxygen and carbon dioxide exchange at the capillary level, while muscle maximally extracts oxygen from the blood, widening the arteriovenous oxygen difference $(C(a-v)_{O2})$.

Procedural Aspects of CPX Testing

Equipment

Similar to standard exercise ECG testing, for CPX exercise is usually performed on a motorized treadmill or bicycle ergometer. Treadmill exercise is preferred, as untrained patients performing bicycle ergometry commonly have a lower peak oxygen uptake ($\dot{V}_{O2}$) due to lower extremity fatigue. Bicycle ergometry may be useful in patients with orthopedic limitations, morbid obesity, or gait disturbance. While arm ergometry has been described in exercise ECG testing, its use for CPX testing is limited as most patients are unable to replicate workloads achieved from treadmill driven protocols.

Gas exchange systems capable of measuring O_2 and CO_2 at rest and during exercise are commercially available. Modern systems are able to adjust for atmospheric conditions such as temperature, barometric pressure, humidity, and oxygen concentration in room air. Systems should be calibrated before each use focusing on the O_2 and CO_2 detectors as well as ventilatory volumes and air flow. In addition to calibration, systems should be validated several times per year.

Exercise Protocols

Exercise protocols with large increases in energy requirements between stages (such as the standard Bruce protocol), demonstrate a weaker relationship between peak $\dot{V}_{O2}$ and work rate. Therefore, protocols with modest increases in work rate per stage, such as the Balke and Ware or Naughton ramp protocols, are recommended. Chapter 5 reviews the various exercise protocols.

Protocol selection should be tailored to each individual patient to achieve a fatigue-limited exercise duration of approximately 8–12 minutes. When test duration is less than six minutes, a nonlinear relationship between $\dot{V}_{O2}$ and work rate may occur, while exercise exceeding 12 minutes may result in muscle fatigue prior to the achievement of peak $\dot{V}_{O2}$.

Preparations and Precautions

Preparations and precautions, including supervision, monitoring, complications, and treatment, for CPX testing are similar to those for exercise ECG testing and are reviewed in Chapter 2.

The risk of complications related to CPX testing is low. One study reported a major cardiovascular event rate of less than 0.5/1000 tests. Nonetheless, appropriate healthcare professionals must be present to provide supervision in the unlikely event that a complication arises. Chapter 2 reviews the personnel, equipment, and medications necessary for safely performing exercise testing. It also reviews precautions and preparations necessary to safely perform exercise testing.

Measurements

Respiratory Assessment

Table 9.1 lists some of the respiratory measurements available during CPX testing.

Table 9.1 Respiratory measurements during cardiopulmonary exercise test (CPX) testing.

Maximal aerobic capacity (MAC) (Peak $\dot{V}_{O2}$)
Ventilatory threshold (V_T)
Peak respiratory exchange ratio (RER)
Ventilatory efficiency ($\dot{V}_E$)
Spirometry
Pulse oximetry

Maximal Aerobic Capacity (Peak VO_2)

Peak $\dot{V}_{O2}$ defines the MAC, representing the physiological limitation of the cardiovascular and pulmonary systems and is generally expressed as ml/kg/min. Derived from the Fick principle, Peak $\dot{V}_{O2} = (HR \times SV) \times [C(a\text{-}v)_{O2}]$, where $HR \times SV$ represents the Q and $C(a\text{-}v)_{O2}$ the arteriovenous oxygen difference.

Ventilatory Threshold

The ventilatory threshold (V_T) is the threshold at which the oxygen supply is unable to meet oxygen demand, resulting in a dependence on anaerobic glycolysis to meet energy demands, resulting in lactate production. The V_T occurs at 45–65% of measured peak $\dot{V}_{O2}$ in healthy participants, but can occur at a higher percentage of peak $\dot{V}_{O2}$ in highly trained individuals.

Peak Respiratory Exchange Ratio (RER)

The RER is defined as the ratio between $\dot{V}_{CO2}$ and $\dot{V}_{O2}$ obtained directly from expired respiratory gas.

A peak RER of ≥1.10 is considered to represent excellent effort during CPX testing, while a peak RER of <1.00 is considered to represent a submaximal effort.

While 85% of age-predicted maximal HR typically represents sufficient participant effort, the RER may be a better assessment of effort. For example, subjects that reach a peak RER of ≥1.1 but achieve 85% of age-predicted maximal heart rate are considered to have reached a maximal effort.

Ventilatory Efficiency

The relationship between minute ventilation ($\dot{V}_E$) and carbon dioxide output $\dot{V}_{CO2}$ are tightly coupled during exercise. Ventilatory efficiency is generally measured by the slope of $\dot{V}_E/\dot{V}_{CO2}$; this parameter has high test–retest reliability. Normal valves are less than 30 without modification for age and sex. An abnormal $\dot{V}_E/\dot{V}_{CO2}$ response reflects systemic disease severity.

Pulmonary Function Testing and Pulse Oximetry

Spirometry is typically performed before exercise providing results for vital capacity, forced expiratory volume in 1 second (FEV1) and inspiratory capacity. Pulse oximetry provides a general estimate of blood hemoglobin oxygenation. A decrease of >5% generally represents abnormal exercise-induced hypoxemia, although this can be seen in fit healthy individuals during high intensity exercise, and therefore is not always indicative of underlying pathology.

Cardiovascular Assessment

Exercise ECG Data

Data obtained from the exercise ECG during CPX testing, when combined the gas exchange assessment, provides a comprehensive cardiopulmonary assessment. Data derived from exercise ECG testing is reviewed in Chapter 14.

Hemodynamic Assessment during Exercise

The hemodynamics of exercise, including normal and abnormal HR and BP responses are reviewed in Chapter 14. As previously described, there is an expected increase in HR and systolic blood pressure (SBP) during exercise of approximately 10 bpm and 10 mmHg/MET, respectively. Chronotropic incompetence and exercise-induced-hypotension are associated with increased mortality.

Symptomatic Assessment

Symptomatic assessment during exercise is reviewed in detail in Chapter 14.

- Symptoms such as fatigue and dyspnea are common.
- Chest pain can occur during exercise and may be similar or dissimilar to index chest pain.
- Typical angina, reproducible with exertion, is predictive of underlying CAD.
- Severe dyspnea, marked pallor, cyanosis, syncope, or near syncope are abnormal responses to exercise.

Applications in Clinical Practice

Heart Failure

CPX testing has multiple applications in patients with HF. At this time, use of CPX testing for the diagnosis of HF is not recommended.

Interestingly, some patients with HF develop a distinct ventilatory pattern with exercise. Referred to as exercise oscillatory ventilation (EOV) or exercise oscillatory breathing (EOB), this is a pathological phenomenon consisting of regular waxing and waning of ventilation (hyperpnea and hypopnea) associated with changes in arterial O_2 and CO_2, which can be detected by CPX testing.

Diagnostic Applications

- Detection of left-sided pulmonary hypertension in patients with HF with reduced and preserved ejection fraction.

Prognostic Recommendations

- Patients with a peak $\dot{V}_{O2}$ of ≤ 14 ml/kg/min, have a higher one-year mortality when compared to those with a peak $\dot{V}_{O2} > 14$ ml/kg/min.
- In patients being considered for cardiac transplantation, advanced mechanical circulatory support, or end stage surgical management, CPX testing is recommended.
- The International Society for Heart Lung Transplantation suggests a peak $\dot{V}_{O2}$ of ≤ 14 ml/kg/min in the absence of a beta-blocker (≤ 12 ml/kg/min with beta-blocker) as an indication for transplant listing.
- In patients with heart failure with reduced ejection fraction (HFrEF), primary CPX variables including $\dot{V}_{E}/\dot{V}_{CO2}$ slope, peak $\dot{V}_{O2}$ and EOV have been shown to be predictors of adverse events. The combination of $\dot{V}_{E}/\dot{V}_{CO2}$ slope ≥ 45.0, peak $\dot{V}_{O2} \leq 10$ ml/kg/min and the presence of EOV carries a poor prognosis.
- Secondary CPX variables have also been shown to be predictors of adverse events in patient with HFrEF.
- $\dot{V}_{E}/\dot{V}_{CO2}$ slope, peak $\dot{V}_{O2}$, and EOV can be useful in providing prognostic information in patients with HF with preserved EF (HFpEF).

Therapy Optimization

- Primary CPX variables, including $\dot{V}_{E}/\dot{V}_{CO2}$ slope, and peak $\dot{V}_{O2}$ can respond to pharmacological, surgical and exercise interventions, and therefore are recommended in guiding therapy in patients with HFrEF. These variables may also be useful in assessing therapy in patients with HFpEF.
- EOV can reverse among patients with HFrEF after pharmacotherapy and exercise interventions.

Unexplained Dyspnea

Dyspnea is a frequent complaint evaluated by healthcare practitioners. When the etiology of dyspnea is not delineated by the combination of a thorough history and physical exam with basic laboratory and diagnostic data, CPX testing may be helpful in distinguishing between cardiovascular and ventilatory limitations to exercise. CPX findings in cardiovascular and pulmonary limitations to exercise are outlined in Table 9.2.

Table 9.2 Cardiopulmonary exercise test (CPX) findings in cardiovascular and pulmonary limitations to exercise.

	Cardiovascular	Pulmonary
Peak $\dot{V}O_2$	Reduced	Reduced
Ventilatory threshold	Reduced	Normal or reduced
$\Delta\dot{V}O_2/\Delta WR$	Often reduced	Normal
Peak HR	May be reduced	May be reduced
Peak $\dot{V}O_2/HR$	Often reduced	May be reduced
Breathing reserve, $1 - (\text{peak } \dot{V}_E/MVV)$	>20%	<15%
Post-exercise FEV_1	Unchanged from rest	May decrease from rest
PaO_2 or SaO_2	Normal	Often reduced
V_D/tidal volume or $\dot{V}_E/\dot{V}CO_2$	May be elevated	Often elevated

MVV, maximum voluntary ventilation; WR, work rate.
Source: Reproduced with permission from: Balady et al. (2010).

Cardiovascular limitations to exercise are characterized by the inability of the cardiovascular system to supply oxygen to meet the demand at a required work rate. As a result, peak $\dot{V}_{O2}$ and ventilatory threshold are typically low.

Ventilatory limitations to exercise are characterized by the inability of the respiratory system to supply oxygen to meet the demands of the body at a required work rate. This may be related to disturbances in ventilation within the lungs or disturbances in diffusion/gas exchange at the alveolar level. Ventilatory limits are identified by a reduction in breathing reserve due to peak $\dot{V}_E$ representing a higher proportion of maximum voluntary ventilation. Diffusion limitations due to ventilation-perfusion (V:Q) mismatch are highlighted by an increased dead space fraction (V_D/tidal volume), which can be measured directly using the Bohr equation. When blood sampling is not available, a high $\dot{V}_E/\dot{V}_{CO2}$ and hypoxemia on pulse oximetry is suggestive of high V_D/tidal volume.

Differentiating cardiovascular and pulmonary limitations to exercise with CPX testing is outlined in Figure 9.1.

Hypertrophic Cardiomyopathy

CPX testing has been helpful in the risk stratification of patients with hypertrophic cardiomyopathy. A recent study of 156 patients with hypertrophic cardiomyopathy undergoing CPX testing with echocardiographic imaging found three independent variables (peak $\dot{V}_{O2}$ <80%, $\dot{V}_E/\dot{V}_{CO2}$ slope >34, and left atrial volume index >40 ml/m^2) associated with an increased risk of death, heart transplantation, and hospitalization for septal reduction.

Other Applications

CPX testing has several emerging applications including:

- Characterization of pulmonary hypertension.
- Assessment of valvular heart disease.

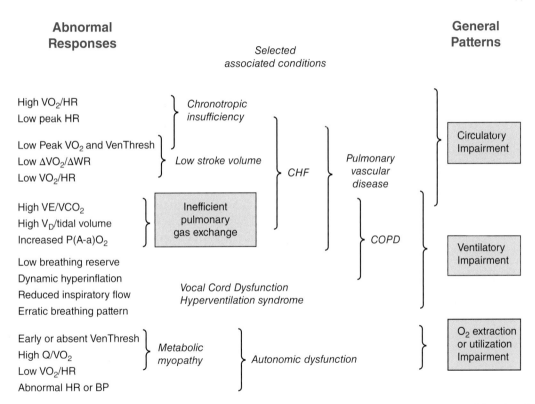

Figure 9.1 Abnormal patterns of responses from cardiopulmonary exercise test (CPX) characteristic of disorders that cause dyspnea. CHF, congestive heart failure; COPD, chronic obstructive pulmonary disease. *Source:* Reproduced, with permission from: Balady et al. (2010).

- Assessment of exercise tolerance and prognosis in patients adult congenital heart disease.
- Optimization of rate-response pacemakers in active patients.
- Assessment of perioperative morbidity and mortality related to lung resection and bariatric surgery.
- Assessment of patients with mitochondrial myopathies.
- Development of an exercise prescription in patients with cardiovascular disease and stroke.

Reporting

Despite a growing body of evidence for the utility of CPX testing, its adoption in clinical practice has been slow. One of the criticisms of CPX testing has been the complexity of data reporting which historically included a large number of variables. In an effort to simplify CPX variable reporting, the European Association for Cardiovascular Prevention & Rehabilitation (EACPR) and the American Heart Association (AHA) have suggested that the reporting of CPX testing focus on clinically relevant variables in a format accessible to referring providers. A sample universal CPX reporting form can be found in published Scientific Statements from the EACPR and AHA.

Summary

- Aerobic exercise represents a balance between the cardiovascular and respiratory systems' ability to supply oxygen to meet the metabolic demands of the body.
- To meet the metabolic demands of the body during exercise, the respiratory system increases oxygen supply by increasing minute ventilation.
- The cardiovascular system increases Q and augments peripheral vasodilation to allow for greater oxygen and carbon dioxide exchange to meet the metabolic demands of the body during exercise.

- Aerobic exercise capacity is an important predictor of adverse events across a wide spectrum of patient populations. One meta-analysis reported a 13% decrease in all-cause mortality and 15% decrease in cardiovascular events for each 1-MET increase in MAC.
- CPX testing allows for a comprehensive assessment of the cardiovascular and respiratory systems during exercise.
- CPX testing is usually performed on a motorized treadmill or bicycle ergometer. Protocols with a moderate increase in work rate per stage, such as the Balke and Ware or Naughton protocols are preferred. Protocols should be tailored to individual patients to achieve a fatigue-limited exercise duration of approximately 8–12 minutes.
- In addition to data obtained from the exercise ECG stress test (with or without myocardial imaging) and spirometry, CPX testing provides an assessment of MAC, ventilatory threshold, peak RER, and ventilatory efficiency.
- CPX testing is well studied in patients with HFrEF and carries important prognostic information: Patients with a peak $\dot{V}_{O2}$ of ≤14 ml/kg/min have a higher 1-year mortality when compared to those with a peak $\dot{V}_{O2}$ >10 ml/kg/min.
- The International Society for Heart Lung Transplantation suggests a peak $\dot{V}_{O2}$ of ≤14 ml/kg/min in the absence of a beta-blocker (≤12 ml/kg/min with beta-blocker) as an indication for heart transplant listing.
- CPX testing can also be helpful in the assessment of unexplained dyspnea.
- Several emerging applications for CPX testing exist.

References

Balady, G.J., Arena, R., Sietsema, K. et al., on behalf of the American Heart Association Exercise, Cardiac Rehabilitation, and Prevention Committee of the Council on Clinical Cardiology; Council on Epidemiology and Prevention; Council on Peripheral Vascular Disease; and Interdisciplinary Council Quality of Care and Outcomes Research (2010). Clinician's guide to cardiopulmonary exercise testing in adults: a scientific statement from the American Heart Association. *Circulation* 122: 191–225.

Finocchiaro, G., Haddad, F., Knowles, J.W. et al. (2015). Cardiopulmonary responses and prognosis in hypertrophic cardiomyopathy: a potential role for comprehensive noninvasive hemodynamic assessment. *J. Am. Coll. Cardiol. Heart Fail.* 3: 408–418.

Fletcher, G.F., Ades, P.A., Kligfield, P. et al., on behalf of the American Heart Association Exercise, Cardiac Rehabilitation, and Prevention Committee of the Council on Clinical Cardiology, Council on Nutrition, Physical Activity and Metabolism, Council on Cardiovascular and Stroke Nursing, and Council on Epidemiology and Prevention (2013). Exercise standards for testing and training: a scientific statement from the American Heart Association. *Circulation* 128: 873–934.

Guazzi, M., Adams, V., Conraads, V. et al., European Association for Cardiovascular Prevention & Rehabilitation; American Heart Association (2012). EACPR/AHA scientific statement: clinical recommendations for cardiopulmonary exercise testing data assessment in specific patient populations. *Circulation* 126: 2261–2274.

Guazzi, M., Arena, R., Halle, M. et al. (2016). Focused update: clinical recommendations for cardiopulmonary exercise testing data assessment in specific patient populations. *Circulation* 133: e694–e711.

Guazzi, M., Bandera, F., Ozemek, C. et al. (2017). Cardiopulmonary exercise testing: what is its value? *J. Am. Coll. Cardiol.* 70: 1618–1636.

Keteyian, S.J., Isaac, D., Thadani, U. et al. (2009). HF-ACTION investigators. Safety of symptom-limited cardiopulmonary exercise testing in patients with chronic heart failure due to severe left ventricular systolic dysfunction. *Am. Heart J.* 158: S72–S77.

Kodama, S., Saito, K., Tanaka, S. et al. (2009). Cardiorespiratory fitness as a quantitative predictor of all-cause mortality and cardiovascular events in healthy men and women: a meta-analysis. *JAMA* 301: 2024–2035.

Miyamura, M. and Honda, Y. (1972). Oxygen intake and cardiac output during maximal treadmill and bicycle exercise. *J. Appl. Physiol.* 32: 185–188.

10 Stress Testing After Acute Coronary Syndromes

Dennis A. Tighe

Introduction

As strategies to treat acute coronary syndromes (ACS), including ST-segment elevation myocardial infarction (STEMI) and non-ST elevation acute coronary syndromes (NSTE-ACS), have evolved so has the approach to the indications for stress testing after these acute coronary events. Much of the currently available clinical data on post-ACS stress testing was collected in the era prior to aggressive therapy of acute myocardial infarction (MI) with thrombolytic agents or percutaneous coronary intervention. With current practice, data suggests that the vast majority of patients with ACS are deemed to be at high-risk and should be treated with an aggressive upfront invasive strategy consisting of early intervention and indicated revascularization. For those patients initially treated with a conservative strategy, the primary role of stress testing remains the identification of the high-risk patient with inducible myocardial ischemia and/or left ventricular (LV) dysfunction in whom further diagnostic evaluation and therapy is indicated. In addition, and equally important, is identification of very low risk sub-groups post-ACS who require little or no further diagnostic evaluation and for whom early return to normal

Pocket Guide to Stress Testing, Second Edition. Edited by Dennis A. Tighe and Bryon A. Gentile.
© 2020 John Wiley & Sons Ltd. Published 2020 by John Wiley & Sons Ltd.

physical activity and occupation can be anticipated. This chapter reviews the data concerning indications for post-ACS stress testing.

Guidelines for Stress Testing After ACS

- As patients presenting to hospital with ACS can be classified into those with STEMI versus NSTE-ACS, guidelines pertaining to the application of stress testing in patients with these two acute syndromes are somewhat different.
- Common to the use of stress testing in both groups is the identification of myocardial ischemia among those who did not initially undergo coronary angiography and detection of residual ischemia/myocardial viability for those not fully revascularized. In addition, an exercise ECG test permits assessment of exercise capacity as part of the cardiac rehabilitation exercise prescription.

Patients with STEMI

- Patients who present to hospital within the 12-hour time window for reperfusion should receive urgent reperfusion therapy and are not considered as candidates for stress testing.
- A non-invasive test, most often resting surface echocardiography, for assessment of LV ejection fraction (EF) and right ventricular function is indicated in all patients.
- Patients who present to hospital after this 12-hour time window and remain hemodynamically stable for >48 hours, defined as no ongoing myocardial ischemia, heart failure (HF), hemodynamic instability, life-threating arrhythmias, or reduced LV EF (<40%) can be considered for stress testing (with or without myocardial imaging) to identify residual myocardial ischemia and for further risk stratification.

- For patients who have not had coronary angiography and do not have high-risk clinical features, stress testing to assess the presence and extent of residual myocardial ischemia is indicated by current ACCF/AHA STEMI guidelines as a Class I, level of evidence B indication.
- Stress testing prior to hospital discharge may also by employed to evaluate the functional significance of a stenotic lesion identified previously at angiography and to guide the post-discharge exercise prescription; both indications are considered to be Class IIb, level of evidence C recommendations.
- Among selected patients identified on clinical grounds as being very low-risk, some centers elect to not perform a pre-discharge submaximal exercise stress test. Instead, a full symptom-limited exercise ECG test is performed three weeks after discharge.
- In patients with non-infarct artery disease who have had successful revascularization of the infarct-related artery and an uncomplicated hospital course, stress imaging can be performed at three to six weeks after discharge.
- The complication rate of post-MI stress testing is low, but somewhat higher than that in patients not having suffered a recent MI (0.02% mortality and 0.05% morbidity).
  Absolute contraindications to post-STEMI stress testing include:
  - Time from MI to testing less than two days.
  - Recurrent myocardial ischemia.
  - Uncontrolled HF within 48–72 hours.
  - Complex ventricular arrhythmia >48 hours post-MI.
  - Uncontrolled hypertension.
  - Severe aortic stenosis.
  - Acute pericarditis or myocarditis.
  - Acute pulmonary embolism/infarction.
- Patients unable to perform stress testing following uncomplicated STEMI constitute a higher risk group.

- In the thrombolytic era, the six-month mortality among patients able perform a stress test is 1–2%, whereas mortality is reported to be 7% among those unable to perform a stress test.
- Both symptom-limited (maximal) and submaximal (low-level) exercise stress testing protocols have been evaluated as pre-discharge testing following STEMI.
- In general, submaximal protocols have been more extensively evaluated, but maximal testing in stable patients has been shown to be safe. When indicated, we usually employ the submaximal test using the modified Bruce protocol in our laboratory.
- Patients should be free of angina pectoris and HF for two to three days prior to performing stress testing.
- Patients unable to perform an exercise ECG test can safely undergo pharmacological stress testing either with vasodilator agents or dobutamine. The same indications and precautions used to select patients for exercise testing also should be applied to those patients considered for pharmacological stress testing.
- Myocardial imaging is required in the 20–30% of patients in whom baseline ECG abnormalities will interfere with interpretation of the ST-segment response to exercise. Imaging is always required when pharmacological stress testing is performed.
- Some centers routinely employ myocardial imaging (stress echocardiography, myocardial perfusion imaging, positron emission tomographic (PET) imaging, or cardiac magnetic resonance) in all patients, regardless of the appearance of their baseline ECG.
- Beta-blocker therapy lowers both resting and exercise heart rate (HR) and systolic blood pressure (SBP). The incidence of exercise-induced angina pectoris and ST-segment depression is also reduced among patients receiving β-blockers. Therefore, the sensitivity of submaximal exercise testing to detect myocardial ischemia is lowered among patients receiving β-blockers.
- In addition to the ECG response to exercise (ST-segment deviation, arrhythmia), other important parameters to be assessed include the hemodynamic response (duration of exercise, SBP rise, HR response) and symptoms elicited (chest pain, dyspnea, fatigue, lightheadedness) during exercise and the results of myocardial imaging

(if obtained). All parameters taken together will determine the functional status of the patient and impart both short- and long-term prognostic implications.

- A recognized limitation to the prognostic value of post-MI stress testing in the current era of early reperfusion is that the predictive accuracy of a positive test for mortality is low. The strongest predictors of death and re-infarction from the exercise ECG stress test are the exercise capacity and the hemodynamic response to exercise.

Patients with NSTE-ACS

- Patients with NSTE-ACS are a more heterogeneous group than those with STEMI. Among patients presenting to an emergency department for evaluation of chest pain, only approximately 5–10% will have ST-segment elevation on ECG, about 15–20% will have a NSTEMI, 10% will have unstable angina pectoris, and upwards of 50% will have non-cardiac disease. Early risk stratification with established clinical risk prediction tools can readily identify groups with high-risk status for whom an early invasive strategy is indicated and a low-risk group for whom an early conservative strategy may be appropriate.
- Similar to patients with STEMI, NSTE-ACS patients with high-risk features should not be referred for stress testing; coronary angiography is indicated for these patients.
- For patients admitted to hospital, a non-invasive test, most often resting surface echocardiography, is indicated for assessment of regional and global LV function.
- Among low-risk NSTE-ACS patients managed with an initial conservative strategy, either a delayed (invasive) strategy or an ischemia-driven strategy can be used.
- When an ischemia-driven strategy is followed, it has been demonstrated that stress testing can be performed safely in patients presenting with unstable angina in 12–24 hours and in 2–5 days among those with NSTEMI, provided that they have remained asymptomatic and show no other high-risk features (Class I indication; level of evidence B).

- Similar to patients undergoing stress testing after STEMI, the choice of stress testing modality should be driven by patient characteristics and local expertise. In general, an exercise ECG (with or without myocardial imaging) should be conducted in patients capable of performing sufficient exercise as significant additional prognostic information is obtained from an exercise bout. Whether or not to perform myocardial imaging in patients with resting ECGs that are interpretable for ST-segment shifts remains controversial; the most recent AHA/ACC guideline statement does not endorse one particular recommendation in this situation; however, the most recent ESC guideline for management of ACS without persistent ST-segment elevation states myocardial imaging is "preferable" for this indication.

Exercise ECG Protocols After ACS

A variety of strategies and exercise ECG protocols can be used to evaluate patients following ACS. As stated above, high-risk patients identified on clinical grounds should not undergo stress testing and are more appropriately evaluated with coronary angiography.

- The strategy most often employed is to perform a submaximal (low-level) exercise ECG test at two to five days post-ACS and just prior to anticipated hospital dismissal in clinically appropriate patients.
- The modified Bruce protocol is most commonly used, but some laboratories prefer the modified Naughton protocol.
- Regardless of the protocol used, the submaximal post-ACS exercise ECG stress test is limited to 70% of age-predicted maximal HR (generally 120–130 bpm) and a workload not exceeding 5–7 metabolic equivalents (METs) depending upon patient age and conditioning.

- An ischemic or high-risk response is an indication for coronary angiography. A "negative" test implies that the patient is safe to be discharged home with a follow-up symptom-limited exercise ECG test to be performed within three to six weeks.
- An alternative strategy is to discharge the clinically very low risk patient (defined as no further chest discomfort, normal or non-diagnostic initial and follow-up ECGs, and normal cardiac biomarker levels) without performing a stress test. A symptom-limited exercise ECG test (Bruce protocol in our laboratory) is performed on an outpatient basis. For patients seen in a chest-pain unit environment, a follow-up stress test is recommended in 24–72 hours. For patients admitted to hospital for "rule-out" and treated with guideline-directed medical therapy, a follow-up stress test is recommended within three to four weeks. An ischemic response constitutes an indication for coronary angiography. A low-risk exercise ECG test implies an excellent one year prognosis with continuation of medical therapy.
- A third strategy is to perform a symptom-limited (maximal) Bruce protocol exercise ECG stress test in clinically low risk patients prior to hospital discharge. This testing may identify more patents with exercise-induced ST-segment depression and chest pain compared to submaximal testing. A follow-up stress test is not required among patients with low-risk results.
- For patients not able to perform an exercise ECG test, vasodilator or dobutamine infusion tests can be used for risk stratification. Use of these tests soon after recent MI (one to three days) in selected patients has been reported to be safe.

Clinical Parameters Assessed by Exercise ECG Testing After ACS

- The parameters assessed during post-ACS exercise ECG stress testing include the hemodynamic response to stress, exercise capacity, symptoms, and ECG changes.
- It is recognized that none of these parameters are completely specific, but they provide useful information to assess overall cardiac functional status.

- Poor exercise tolerance (<4 METs), an excessive HR response, a decrease in SBP, and ST-segment depression with exercise (particularly when accompanied by symptoms) may be indicative of stress-induced severe impairment of LV function and predictive of an increased risk for future cardiac events.
- Myocardial ischemia during or following stress can produce angina or shortness of breath, and poor ventricular function can cause dyspnea or fatigue. However, these symptoms are not entirely specific and, in particular, the occurrence of angina pectoris shows limited reproducibility and substantial individual variability when a pre-discharge stress test is compared to a later symptom-limited test.

Results of Exercise ECG Testing After MI

- Approximately 60% of patients undergoing treadmill exercise after MI will achieve a workload of 6 METs or a HR of 70% of age-predicted maximal HR without limiting symptoms.
- Approximately 15–40% will experience limiting angina pectoris.
- ST-segment depression will occur in 10–25% of patients.
- Ventricular ectopy will occur in 20–30% of patients.
- The reported incidence of exercise-induced ST-segment elevation is variable. ST-segment elevation almost always occurs in the ECG leads which face the infarcted area.

Prognostic Value of Post-ACS Stress Testing

Hemodynamic Response

- An inadequate increase of SBP above the resting level with exercise implies myocardial ischemia and/or LV dysfunction and is an unfavorable prognostic sign. Although defined variably in the literature, an inadequate BP increase is generally indicated by a ≤ 10–20 mmHg rise in SBP or a peak SBP of ≤ 110 mmHg.

- A decrease in SBP of ≥20 mmHg during exercise is an unfavorable prognostic sign that is predictive of an increased risk of future coronary events.

Exercise Capacity

- In the absence of limiting non-cardiac conditions, the inability to perform a 4 MET workload at three weeks post-ACS often reflects severe LV dysfunction and is predictive of an increased risk of future cardiac events.
- Several studies have demonstrated that exercise capacity is the single most important factor influencing prognosis in the post-ACS population. In one study, for each 1 MET increase in exercise capacity, a 12% improvement in survival was conferred.
- The inability to perform a pre-discharge exercise stress test has been associated with a fivefold higher six-month mortality compared to patients capable of performing an exercise bout.

Angina Pectoris

- Exercise-induced angina occurs in 15–40% of patients undergoing post-ACS exercise ECG testing.
- Some studies indicate that exercise-induced angina is an independent predictor of future cardiac events. However, other investigators have shown that exercise-induced angina is highly predictive of future angina pectoris, but is not an independent predictor of cardiac death.

Stress-Induced ECG Abnormalities
ST-Segment Depression

- Exercise-induced ST-segment depression occurs in about 10–25% of patients undergoing a post-MI exercise ECG test.
- Among patients receiving thrombolytic therapy, the incidence of exercise-induced ST-segment depression is reported to be 50% less than patients who did not receive a thrombolytic agent.

- Exercise-induced ST-segment depression on a submaximal post-MI exercise ECG test is a marker of myocardial ischemia and may be useful prognostic sign in patients following acute MI.
  - Patients who develop >1 mm of ST-segment depression have an increased risk of cardiac death compared to patients with a normal ST-segment response. In the era prior to acute reperfusion, a 13-fold difference in one-year mortality was observed for patients having an ischemic exercise ECG response.
  - In the era of reperfusion, exercise-induced ST-segment depression after fibrinolytic therapy has been shown to be predictive of death and recurrent infarction; however, this association is not clearly as predicative among those having primary percutaneous coronary intervention.
  - The severity of ST-segment depression correlates, as does its timing, with future cardiac events. The risk of a cardiac event is twofold higher among patients with ST-segment depression ≥2 mm as compared to patients with <2 mm of ST-segment depression. Occurrence of ST-segment depression early in the exercise bout is also associated with adverse prognosis.
- Patients with <2 mm of exercise-induced ST-segment depression and a good exercise workload (≥7 METs) have a favorable prognosis in the absence of exercise-induced angina.
- The presence of resting ST-segment abnormalities (LVH with repolarization abnormality, LBBB, digitalis effect, etc.) reduces the predictive accuracy of exercise-induced ST-segment depression. Myocardial imaging is required in these patients.
- Although ST-segment depression with exercise has been associated with increased risk, several studies have shown that poor exercise capacity and/or abnormal hemodynamic response to stress to be the strongest indicators of adverse prognosis.

ST-Segment Elevation

- Exercise-induced ST-segment elevation following recent MI is a non-specific sign, which most frequently occurs in the ECG leads which reflect the infarcted area.

- Most investigators believe that stress-induced ST-segment elevation in leads which correspond to the area of MI primarily represents LV dysfunction and abnormal wall motion in the infarct zone.
- Exercise-induced ST-segment elevation in leads other than the infarct zone (excluding leads aVR and V1) may represent transmural myocardial ischemia.

Exercise-Induced Ventricular Arrhythmia

- The prognostic significance of ventricular arrhythmia during post-ACS exercise ECG testing remains controversial.
- Ventricular ectopy occurs in up to 30% of patients during post-ACS stress testing.
- Some investigators believe that exercise-induced ventricular arrhythmia is predictive of future cardiac events while other groups have shown it to have little prognostic value.
- Overall it appears that exercise-induced ventricular ectopy as independent factor is not as predictive of future cardiac events compared to factors such as stress-induced angina, ST-segment depression, hypotension, and low exercise workload.
- Ventricular ectopy during exercise appears to be a marker of underlying myocardial ischemia and/or LV dysfunction.

Myocardial Imaging

- Myocardial imaging, with nuclear perfusion agents or echocardiography, in conjunction with the post-ACS exercise ECG test, is indicated when pre-existing ECG abnormalities or medication use may interfere with interpretation of the ST-segment response to exercise. Some professional guidelines recommend the routine use of myocardial imaging in all patients having a post-ACS stress test.

- In addition to improved accuracy to diagnose residual ischemia compared to the exercise ECG stress test, myocardial imaging permits localization of residual ischemia, assessment of extent of disease (single versus multivessel disease), and identification of viable myocardium. Estimation of resting and stress-induced LV EF can be obtained with echocardiography and radionuclide ventriculography (RVG).
- Early studies with gated RVG showed that imaging (non-exercise) parameters, such as resting LVEF, LV volumes, and EF response to exercise (<5% increase or >5% decrease in EF with stress), were associated with adverse prognosis in post-MI patients. Exercise RVG has now been supplanted by imaging with gated rest/stress SPECT myocardial perfusion imaging and echocardiography for risk stratification.
- Thallium-201 scintigraphy has been the most widely studied myocardial imaging technique for post-MI stress testing; however abundant data for 99m-Technetium myocardial perfusion scintigraphy and echocardiography exist. Among post-MI patients who underwent exercise-ECG testing with concomitant myocardial perfusion imaging (MPI), parameters independent of exercise data identified as strong predictors of future cardiac events include:
  - Presence of transient (reversible) perfusion defects in the infarct zone or in another vessel territory (remote ischemia)
  - Extent of perfusion defects
  - Increased lung uptake of ^{201}Th after stress
  - Stress-induced (transient) LV cavity dilatation
  - Degree of LV dysfunction as assessed by LVEF (<40%)
- Patients without these adverse findings on MPI have an excellent one-year prognosis. Some studies have demonstrated that exercise-MPI is more predictive of future cardiac events than is coronary angiography.
- Among patients who receive thrombolytic therapy and undergo post-MI exercise MPI, redistribution of radiotracer is present significantly more often than is exercise-induced ST-segment depression.
- Pharmacological stress-MPI with vasodilator agents has been studied extensively in the post-MI population. Similar to exercise-MPI data, identification of scintigraphic ischemia, the extent of perfusion defects and the LVEF

are predictors of adverse cardiac events. A particularly high-risk group is characterized by a $\geq 20\%$ total LV perfusion defect size with $>10\%$ ischemia and reduced LVEF. Conversely, a low-risk group with small perfusion defect size ($<20\%$), minimal ischemia ($<10\%$) and preserved LVEF can be identified.

- A number of studies have evaluated the use of exercise or pharmacological stress echocardiography following a recent MI.
  - During exercise echocardiography, the occurrence of new or worsening wall motion abnormalities identifies patients with increased risk of future cardiac events more reliably than does exercise-induced ST-segment depression. The extent and severity of new wall motion abnormality correlates directly with prognosis. Dysynergy during stress in a vascular supply region different from the infarct territory and/or LV cavity dilatation is indicative of multivessel disease. Among post-MI patients without such exercise-induced findings, the risk of future cardiac events is low.
  - With pharmacological stress echocardiography (dobutamine or vasodilator agents), various investigators have shown that worsening of regional wall motion within the infarct zone during stress is indicative of ischemia and new wall motion abnormality outside of the region of infarction indicates the presence of multi-vessel disease. In addition to the extent and severity of ischemia (wall motion score index), some studies have reported that a positive response at a low infusion dose is associated with worse outcomes than when such a response occurred at higher-infused doses. High-risk findings include reduced resting LVEF ($<40\%$), extensive ischemia (≥ 5 wall segments) induced by stress, large infarction size (≥ 5 wall segments), reduction of LVEF from rest to stress, and occurrence of LV cavity dilation with stress.
  - In addition to identifying stress-induced ischemia, dobutamine stress echocardiography can be used to assess for myocardial viability in the infarct zone (presence of residual coronary stenosis). Improved contractility during low dose dobutamine infusion (2.5–10 mcg/kg/min) with deterioration of function at higher doses, the so-called "biphasic response", is a specific finding suggesting the presence of viable myocardium.

Summary

- The majority of clinical data available regarding the post-ACS exercise ECG test was collected in the era prior to urgent reperfusion therapy of acute MI.
- For those patients treated with an initial conservative strategy and who remain clinically stable, the goal of post-ACS stress testing is the identification of the high-risk patient with inducible myocardial ischemia/viability and/or LV dysfunction.
- Patients with recurrent myocardial ischemia, uncontrolled HF, or electrical instability are at high-risk and should not be referred for stress testing. Patients with these characteristics should more appropriately be referred for coronary angiography.
- Exercise testing offers more functional information and has been more extensively studied as compared to pharmacological stress imaging. However, pharmacological stress agents have been safely and effectively used in patients following recent ACS for risk stratification.
- As with routine exercise testing, the combination of clinical variables, exercise-induced ECG and hemodynamic alterations, and exercise capacity offers superior prognostic information in comparison to reliance on a single variable.
- High-risk patients during post-ACS exercise ECG stress testing include those with inducible ischemia at a low workload, poor exercise capacity, exercise-induced angina, blunted HR response, and impaired BP with exercise. Those unable to perform a stress test constitute a very high-risk group.
- Nuclear myocardial perfusion abnormalities associated with poor prognosis include the number and location of reversible perfusion defect(s), presence of reduced LVEF, transient ischemic dilatation of the LV cavity, and increased lung uptake of radiotracer after stress. Similarly with echocardiography, the extent of inducible myocardial ischemia, occurrence of LV cavity dilatation with stress, and/or a reduction in LVEF are associated with adverse prognosis.

- Patients identified as being at high-risk, and most patients at intermediate risk, based on the findings of post-ACS stress testing should be referred for coronary angiography.
- Conversely, low-risk patients often do not require coronary angiography. Appropriate use of guideline-directed medical therapy and close clinical follow-up for recurrent symptoms is indicated. If a submaximal ECG stress test was performed prior to discharge, a maximal test is indicated at three to six weeks post ACS.

References

American College of Emergency Physicians; Society for Cardiovascular Angiography and Interventions, O'Gara, P.T., Kushner, F.G. et al. (2013). ACCF/AHA guideline for the management of ST-elevation myocardial infarction: a report of the American College of Cardiology Foundation/American Heart Association Task Force on Practice Guidelines. *J. Am. Coll. Cardiol.* 61: e78–e140.

Amsterdam, E.A., Kirk, J.D., Bluemke, D.A. et al., American Heart Association Exercise, Cardiac Rehabilitation, and Prevention Committee of the Council on Clinical Cardiology, Council on Cardiovascular Nursing, and Interdisciplinary Council on Quality of Care and Outcomes Research (2010). Testing of low-risk patients presenting to the emergency department with chest pain: a scientific statement from the American Heart Association. *Circulation* 122: 1756–1776.

Amsterdam, E.A., Wenger, N.K., Brindis, R.G. et al. (2014). 2014 AHA/ACC Guideline for the Management of Patients with Non-ST-Elevation Acute Coronary Syndromes: a report of the American College of Cardiology/American Heart Association Task Force on Practice Guidelines. *J. Am. Coll. Cardiol.* 64: e139–e228.

Bigi, R., Cortigiani, L., Desideri, A. et al. (2001). Clinical and angiographic correlates of dobutamine-induced wall motion patterns after myocardial infarction. *Am. J. Cardiol.* 88: 944–948.

Dakik, H.A., Wendt, J.A., Kimball, K. et al. (2005). Prognostic value of adenosine Tl-201 myocardial perfusion imaging after acute myocardial infarction: results of a prospective clinical trial. *J. Nucl. Cardiol.* 12: 276–283.

Hoedemaker, N.P.G., Damman, P., Woudstra, P. et al. (2017). Early invasive versus selective strategy for non-ST-segment elevation acute coronary syndrome: the ICTUS trial. *J. Am. Coll. Cardiol.* 69: 1883–1893.

Ibanez, B., James, S., Agewall, S. et al., ESC Scientific Document Group (2018). 2017 ESC guidelines for the management of acute myocardial infarction in patients presenting with ST-segment elevation: the task force for the management of acute myocardial infarction in patients presenting with ST-segment elevation of the European Society of Cardiology (ESC). *Eur. Heart J.* 39: 119–177.

Kavanagh, T., Mertens, D.J., Hamm, L.F. et al. (2002). Prediction of long-term prognosis in 12 169 men referred for cardiac rehabilitation. *Circulation* 106: 666–671.

Mahmarian, J.J., Dwivedi, G., Lahiri, T. et al. (2004). Role of nuclear cardiac imaging in myocardial infarction: postinfarction risk stratification. *J. Nucl. Cardiol.* 11: 186–209.

Mahmarian, J.J., Shaw, L.J., Filipchuk, N.G. et al., INSPIRE Investigators (2006). A multinational study to establish the value of early adenosine technetium-99m sestamibi myocardial perfusion imaging in identifying a low-risk group for early hospital discharge after acute myocardial infarction. *J. Am. Coll. Cardiol.* 48: 2448–2457.

Myers, J., Prakash, M., Froelicher, V. et al. (2002). Exercise capacity and mortality among men referred for exercise testing. *N. Engl. J. Med.* 346: 793–801.

Roffi, M., Patrono, C., Collet, J.P. et al., ESC Scientific Document Group (2016). 2015 ESC guidelines for the management of acute coronary syndromes in patients presenting without persistent ST-segment elevation: Task Force for the Management of Acute Coronary Syndromes in Patients Presenting without Persistent ST-Segment Elevation of the European Society of Cardiology (ESC). *Eur. Heart J.* 37: 267–315.

Shaw, L.J., Peterson, E.D., Kesler, K. et al. (1996). A meta-analysis of predischarge risk stratification after acute myocardial infarction with stress electrocardiographic, myocardial perfusion, and ventricular function imaging. *Am. J. Cardiol.* 78: 1327–1337.

Sicari, R., Landi, P., Picano, E. et al., EPIC (Echo Persantine International Cooperative); EDIC (Echo Dobutamine International Cooperative) Study Group (2002). Exercise-electrocardiography and/or pharmacological stress echocardiography for non-invasive risk stratification early after uncomplicated myocardial infarction. A prospective international large scale multicentre study. *Eur. Heart J.* 23: 1030–1037.

Valeur, N., Clemmensen, P., Saunamäki, K., and Grande, P., DANAMI-2 investigators (2005). The prognostic value of pre-discharge exercise testing after myocardial infarction treated with either primary PCI or fibrinolysis: a DANAMI-2 sub-study. *Eur. Heart J.* 26: 119–127.

Villella, A., Maggioni, A.P., Villella, M. et al. (1995). Prognostic significance of maximal exercise testing after myocardial infarction treated with thrombolytic agents: the GISSI-2 data-base. Gruppo Italiano per lo Studio della Sopravvivenza Nell'Infarto. *Lancet* 346: 523–529.

11   Proper Selection of the Mode of Stress Testing

Dennis A. Tighe

Introduction

Non-invasive functional cardiac assessment provides important diagnostic and prognostic information in patients with suspected or known cardiovascular disease and its results can be used to guide and monitor therapy. To achieve these goals, clinicians have at their disposal a number and variety of methods to perform cardiac stress testing. Previous chapters have described these methods, the various stress testing protocols available, and test interpretation in detail. In addition a complete discussion of false positive and false negative exercise ECG test results can be found in Chapter 15. This chapter will review indications, limitations, and selection of a specific mode of stress testing and possible associated imaging technique to optimize diagnostic and prognostic information for the individual patient.

Pocket Guide to Stress Testing, Second Edition. Edited by Dennis A. Tighe and Bryon A. Gentile.
© 2020 John Wiley & Sons Ltd. Published 2020 by John Wiley & Sons Ltd.

General Comments

- Prior to requesting a particular type of stress test, the referring provider must clearly determine:
  - The goal of the stress test (diagnosis of coronary artery disease [CAD], exercise capacity, assessing prognosis, efficacy of medical or surgical therapy, localizing ischemia, assessing myocardial viability, etc.).
  - If contraindications to stress testing exist (see Chapter 4)
  - Limitations of a particular method.
  - Potential for false-positive or false-negative results, as based upon available clinical and ECG-related factors.
  - The influence on future management of a divergent result.
- For diagnostic purposes, complete assessment of historical factors (age, gender, type and nature of chest pain, cardiac risk factors), a full clinical evaluation of the patient, appreciation that pre-test risk of disease is related to the prevalence of that disease in the population studied (Table 11.1), and understanding of the concepts of test sensitivity, specificity, and predicative accuracy are important for proper interpretation of the test's results.
- Consideration of the principles of Bayes' theorem, which incorporates the pre-test risk of disease (based on known clinical factors) and the sensitivity and specificity of the test (likelihood ratio) to calculate post-test probability of disease, is warranted because it is appreciated that stress ECG results should be interpreted on a continuum of risk based on extent of ST-segment depression induced by exercise rather than using a strict cut-off of ≥1 mm horizontal or downsloping ST-segment depression to define a test a "positive." The diagnostic yield of the exercise ECG test is maximized when the pre-test likelihood of disease is intermediate (variably defined as 10–90%, 20–80% or 30–70% pre-test likelihood of CAD). Testing of patients with very low or low pre-test risk of disease (<5–10%) is not encouraged due to the high incidence of false positive tests. For patients with high pre-test likelihood of disease (>90%), testing of subjects to diagnose CAD is not recommended as most tests without significant ST-segments shifts will constitute false negative responses. The post-test probability of ischemic heart disease can be estimated

Table 11.1 Pretest probability of coronary artery disease (CAD) according to age, gender, and symptoms.

Age (years)	Gender	Typical/Definite angina pectoris	Atypical/Probable angina pectoris	Nonanginal chest pain	Asymptomatic
<39	Men	Intermediate	Intermediate	Low	Very low
	Women	Intermediate	Very low	Very low	Very low
40–49	Men	High	Intermediate	Intermediate	Low
	Women	Intermediate	Low	Very low	Very low
50–59	Men	High	Intermediate	Intermediate	Low
	Women	Intermediate	Intermediate	Low	Very low
>60	Men	High	Intermediate	Intermediate	Low
	Women	High	Intermediate	Intermediate	Low

Source: Reproduced with permission from: Douglas et al. (2011).
High: >90% pre-test probability; Intermediate: Between 10 and 90% pre-test probability; Low: Between 5 and 10% pre-test probability; Very low: <5% pre-test probability.

from the data of investigators such as Diamond and Forrester, the Duke Database for Cardiovascular Disease, and others. Figure 11.1 illustrates the application of Bayes' theorem to exercise ECG test results among four hypothetical patients with differing pretest likelihood of disease.

- Variables derived from exercise ECG testing beyond just the ST-segment response provide important diagnostic and prognostic information. Use of this information, such as with the Duke treadmill score (DTS) and post-exercise HR recovery, should be considered strongly in recommending therapy and need for further testing. Subjects with low-risk DTS scores, often can be managed initially with medical therapy while those DTS indicating

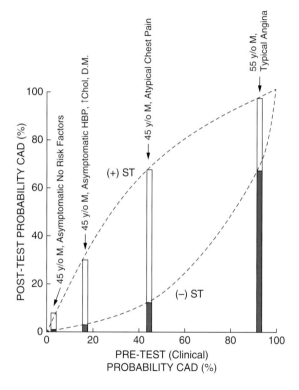

Figure 11.1 Application of Bayes' theorem to estimate the post exercise test probability of coronary artery disease (CAD). The pretest probability of disease (increasing from left to right) based on existing clinical data is displayed on the X-axis. When the clinical data is combined with the ECG response to exercise (positive [+] or negative [–] ST-segment depression), a post-test probability of CAD (increasing along the vertical axis) is obtained. The test is assumed to have a sensitivity of 84% and specificity of 62%. Four specific patient examples are shown by vertical bars, where the height of the solid bar demonstrates the results for an exercise ECG test without ST-segment depression, (–) ST, and the open bar shows the results for a test with ST-segment depression, (+) ST. As illustrated by the example of the third patient from the left, the predictive power of ST-segment depression is highest when the pretest risk of disease is intermediate. ST-segment depression in the patient at the far left, with a very small pretest likelihood of CAD, is much more likely a false positive rather than a true positive result. In contrast, a lack of significant ST-segment depression in a patient, such as the one at the far right, with a high pretest likelihood of CAD is more likely to represent a false negative rather than a true negative response. *Source:* Reproduced with permission from: Patterson and Horowitz (1989). Chol, cholesterol; DM, diabetes mellitus; HBP, high blood pressure; M, male.

high-risk should proceed on to coronary angiography and revascularization as indicated. Patients with intermediate DTS are often best risk-stratified by repeating the exercise stress ECG test with myocardial imaging.

- Pharmacologic stress testing (vasodilators or dobutamine) does not provide the hemodynamic information available from an exercise bout. Because the hemodynamic information available from exercise testing offers significant additional clinical and prognostic data, a stress test that incorporates maximal exercise is the preferred stress testing method whenever possible.
- ST-segment depression during ECG stress testing does not localize the potential area of myocardial ischemia. ST-segment elevation in leads without q-waves, an uncommon occurrence, often indicates the presence of transmural myocardial ischemia that localizes hypoperfusion to the distribution of a particular coronary artery.
- Stress myocardial imaging (myocardial perfusion agents or echocardiography) increases the diagnostic accuracy of the exercise ECG test. Myocardial imaging also has the capability to localize and define the extent of ischemia.
- Stress echocardiography and radionuclide ventriculography (rarely used today) allow direct measurement of the LVEF at rest and its response to stress. A gated, first-pass estimate of LVEF is available with single photon emission computed tomographic (SPECT) or positron emission tomographic (PET) myocardial perfusion imaging.
- Myocardial imaging techniques add significant cost and time compared to the standard exercise ECG stress test. In the case of myocardial perfusion imaging (MPI), patient exposure to ionizing radiation occurs.
- When selecting a mode of stress testing, consideration should include the recommendations made in guideline and appropriate use documents promulgated by various professional societies which provide information on the appropriate use of these modalities in various clinical scenarios.
- The decision to withhold or administer various medications prior to a stress test should be made by the referring provider in accord with the overall goal(s) of the stress test. Most often, anti-anginal medications are withheld prior to testing as they are known to reduce the sensitivity of the test. When the efficacy of a medical regimen is to be assessed, the patient should receive these medicines in full doses up the time of the stress test.

Selection of Mode Stress Testing (see Figure 11.2)

Standard Exercise ECG Stress Test

- The majority of patients with a normal or near-normal resting ECG (≤ 0.5 to 1.0 mm ST-segment depressions) who are not receiving digitalis (a relatively small number of patients receive digitalis in current practice) are potential candidates for a symptom-limited exercise ECG test without myocardial imaging as an initial method for detection of CAD. Most subjects with right bundle branch block can undergo a standard exercise ECG stress test for diagnosis of CAD.
- When considering an exercise ECG test, the clinician should appreciate if the patient has the capability to perform an adequate exercise bout. In general, patients who cannot perform the routine activities of daily living (about four to five metabolic equivalents [METs]) will not likely be able to perform an adequate level of stress for diagnostic purposes and should be referred for pharmacological stress testing. To ascertain the patient's ability to perform an adequate level of stress, we specifically inquire of our patients as to their daily activity levels ("can you climb one to two flights of stairs without stopping?"; "how far can you walk on a flat surface without limitation?"). Questionnaires, such as the Duke Activity Status Index, can be used to provide a more formal assessment of the ability to achieve an adequate exercise workload.
- Among patients with a normal resting ECG and the ability to achieve an adequate exercise workload for age and gender, the sensitivity and specificity of the exercise ECG stress test are sufficiently high enough to detect significant CAD without the need for myocardial imaging techniques. An exception to this initial approach would be the patient with known CAD and prior revascularization for whom we often recommend exercise ECG stress myocardial imaging to localize and define the extent of ischemia.
- Hemodynamic information obtained from the exercise ECG stress test offers valuable diagnostic and prognostic information (see Chapter 17).

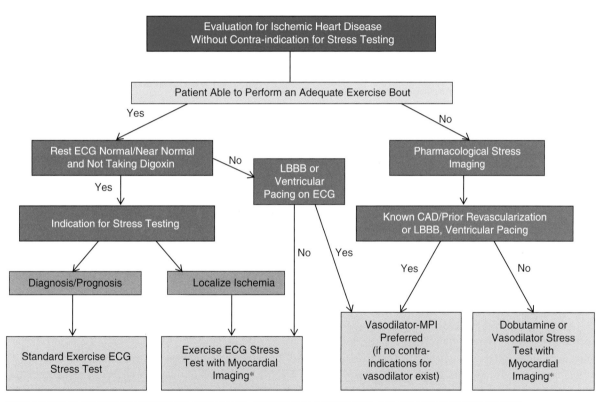

*Base decision on factors that include patient characteristics, local expertise and availability, cost, and ionizing radiation exposure.

Figure 11.2 An algorithm for selecting of a particular type of stress test for an individual patient.

- The exercise ECG test can be performed at a significantly lower cost and in less time than stress tests requiring myocardial imaging.
- The standard ECG stress test may be used in patients with an abnormal resting ECG or in those receiving digitalis if total exercise capacity and the chronotropic or hemodynamic response to exercise, rather than detection of CAD, are the goals of the stress test.

Use of Myocardial Imaging Techniques

- Myocardial imaging techniques are indicated in most patients for whom the diagnostic capability of the standard exercise ECG stress test for detecting CAD is limited.
- Specific situations in which concomitant myocardial imaging is indicated include:
  - Abnormal resting ECG (Wolff-Parkinson-White pattern, left ventricular hypertrophy (LVH) with repolarization abnormality, left bundle branch block (LBBB), non-specific abnormality of the ST-segment and T-wave, ventricular-paced rhythm, hypokalemia with ST-segment abnormality).
  - Digitalis use.
  - Anticipated submaximal exercise workload.
  - Non-diagnostic exercise ECG test results.
  - Intermediate risk DTS.
  - Need to localize ischemia or assess myocardial viability.
  - Pharmacological stress testing.
  - Anti-anginal medicine use (false-negative study).
- Among women, a relatively high incidence of false-positive ST-segment depression during exercise ECG stress testing is reported. To address this issue, the randomized WOMEN trial, which was conducted among symptomatic women with an interpretable ECG and ability to perform an adequate exercise bout, showed that there was

no incremental benefit for an upfront myocardial imaging strategy in two-year clinical outcomes while providing diagnostic cost savings. For symptomatic women with intermediate risk for CAD and an interpretable ECG, the most recent AHA consensus statement recommends an initial strategy of standard exercise ECG testing.

- Myocardial imaging techniques allow localization of ischemic vascular territories and evaluation of the extent of ischemia. Both echocardiography and nuclear MPI are well validated to offer both diagnostic and prognostic information. Among patients known CAD, we preferentially recommend MPI to echocardiography for this purpose.

- The use of a specific imaging technique should be tailored to the individual patient, the method of stress used, and local availability and expertise. In general, MPI is superior to echocardiography when vasodilator infusion is the method of stress, while echocardiography is the preferred method for use in conjunction with dobutamine infusion.

- Echocardiography is the preferred technique when ancillary information such as LVEF and regional wall motion, assessment of the cardiac valves, estimation of the pulmonary artery systolic pressure, and evaluation for pericardial disease is desired.

- Among the nuclear perfusion agents, ^{201}Tl is the most widely investigated agent. Its main advantages include its extensively validated use for detection of myocardial viability and assessment of post-stress lung uptake. The main disadvantage of ^{201}Tl is its low emitted energy which limits image resolution in obese patients with much soft tissue and the greater exposure of the patient to ionizing radiation; primarily for the latter reason, ^{201}Tl is no longer in common use in most laboratories.

- Technetium-based agents (most often used radiotracer today) are superior to ^{201}Tl for use in obese patients and a bolus injection can be used to obtain a first-pass ejection fraction. It appears that 99m Tc agents minimally redistribute, and therefore may be less useful for detecting viable myocardium than is ^{201}Tl.

- Nuclear perfusion agents should be used in the occasional patient in whom adequate transthoracic echocardiographic windows cannot be obtained for stress echocardiography. Some clinicians in this situation may elect to perform dobutamine echocardiography using the transesophageal technique.

- As compared to echocardiography, stress testing utilizing nuclear MPI agents is more costly, the imaging protocols are more time-consuming, and patient exposure to ionizing radiation occurs (a significant concern in younger subjects). In general, the ALARA ("As Low As Reasonably Achievable") principle should be followed to minimize radiation exposure to the patient while still obtaining diagnostic information.

Vasodilator Stress Testing (see Chapter 8)

- Pharmacological stress testing with a vasodilator agent (dipyridamole, adenosine, regadenoson) is indicated for patients unable to achieve an adequate workload during exercise ECG stress testing. Specific situations include peripheral vascular disease, orthopedic limitation, neurological impairment, and other infirmities which limit physical exercise.
- Vasodilator agent use in combination with MPI has been studied extensively in the pre-operative cardiac evaluation of patients prior to vascular surgery.
- Among patients with fixed LBBB or ventricular pacing, the preferred method in most laboratories, including ours, is to assess for myocardial ischemia with vasodilator-MPI due to false positive findings (septal perfusion defects not related to obstructive CAD) that can occur with exercise or dobutamine myocardial perfusion imaging. For patients unable to have a vasodilator-MPI stress test, dobutamine echocardiography is a reasonable alternative method with acceptable diagnostic performance (high specificity, but reduced sensitivity for detection of left anterior descending territory CAD).
- Concomitant myocardial imaging is required with vasodilator stress due to the low sensitivity of ST-segment depression and high incidence of non-specific chest discomfort associated with their use.
- Myocardial perfusion agents appear to be superior to echocardiography as the imaging technique of choice due to the relatively small increase in rate-pressure product accompanying vasodilator infusion.

- Contraindications to the use of the vasodilator agents include:
  - Reactive airways disease (bronchospasm, asthma)
  - Severe obstructive lung disease
  - Active or recently symptomatic cerebrovascular disease
  - Acute myocardial infarction (within 48 hours)
  - Active unstable angina pectoris
  - Severe aortic stenosis
  - Advanced A-V block in the absence of a pacemaker
  - Hypotension
- Patients actively taking oral dipyridamole or medications containing dipyridamole should not receive adenosine or regadenoson infusion due to the risk of advanced AV block and hypotension. Instead, infusion of dobutamine or dipyridamole can be safely employed in these patients.
- Methylxanthine-type medications act as competitive inhibitors of adenosine receptors and interfere with the mechanism of action of vasodilator agents. It is recommended that these medications be withheld for a minimum of 12 hours prior to testing.
- Caffeine (contained in coffee, teas, colas) and medications containing caffeine (many prescription and over-the-counter preparations) should be withheld for a minimum of 12 hours prior to testing to achieve maximal coronary vasodilatation.
- Pentoxifylline, a medication used for the treatment of intermittent claudication among patients with chronic occlusive arterial disease, is pharmacologically related to the xanthine family and may interfere with the action of vasodilator agents. Our practice is to recommend that pentoxifylline be withheld for 36–48 hours prior to anticipated testing or recommend that another form of stress testing (usually dobutamine) be performed.

Dobutamine Stress Testing (see Chapters 7 and 8)

- Chapters 7 and 8 discuss dobutamine stress testing in more detail.
- Dobutamine is a synthetic catecholamine which acts to increase myocardial contractility and HR, thereby leading to an increase in myocardial oxygen demand. As opposed to vasodilator infusion, dobutamine use more closely mimics the hemodynamic response to exercise.
- Dobutamine infusion also requires a concomitant myocardial imaging procedure for maximal diagnostic accuracy.
- Echocardiography is most commonly used; however myocardial perfusion agents can be employed with similar reported sensitivity and specificity.
- The main advantages of dobutamine echocardiography over nuclear perfusion imaging include:
  - Immediate assessment and reporting.
  - Documentation of myocardial ischemia at a particular infusion rate (ability to define an ischemic threshold).
  - Global assessment of LV function at rest and in response to stress.
  - Assessment of other (potentially previously unrecognized) cardiac pathology by echocardiography.
  - Lower cost.
  - Lack of exposure to ionizing radiation.
- Dobutamine infusion is more time-consuming than a stress session with vasodilator or exercise ECG testing. In patients receiving beta-blockers or when the chronotropic effect of dobutamine is blunted, the infusion protocol may take more than 20 minutes to complete.
- Dobutamine use is contraindicated among patients with unstable angina, acute MI within two to four days, uncontrolled hypertension (SBP >200 mmHg and/or DBP >110 mmHg), hemodynamically significant LV outflow tract obstruction, uncontrolled atrial arrhythmia, and when life-threatening ventricular arrhythmias are present. Large or symptomatic abdominal aortic aneurysm may constitute a relative contraindication, but data is somewhat sparse in this regard.

Cardiopulmonary Exercise Testing

- Cardiopulmonary exercise testing (CPX) is discussed in more detail in Chapter 9.
- Cardiopulmonary stress testing is a technique that involves analysis of respiratory expired gas exchange (maximal oxygen uptake, carbon dioxide production, ventilatory threshold, respiratory exchange ratio, and minute ventilation) and monitoring of arterial oxygen saturation. This information is integrated with the standard information obtained during an exercise stress ECG test. Pulmonary function testing can be included for select patients.
- Maximal (peak) VO_2 is measured directly with CPX, rather than estimated as with standard exercise ECG stress testing.
- Treadmill exercise (ramp protocols preferred) or bicycle ergometry are the standard methods of stress. Values for maximal (peak) VO_2 are 10–20% lower with cycle ergometry compared to treadmill exercise. Heart rate and rhythm are monitored continuously and BP is measured periodically throughout the test.
- Indications for CPX are expanding and include evaluation of functional assessment in patients with HF, timing of cardiac transplantation/LV assist device implant, evaluation of unexplained dyspnea (cardiac versus pulmonary limitation), functional assessment of patients with congenital heart disease, and assessment of exercise capacity when indicated for medical reasons when estimates of exercise capacity from exercise test time or work rate are unreliable.
- Serial CPX to measure peak oxygen consumption can be used in the heart failure with reduced ejection fraction (HFrEF) population to assess the response to medical therapy and stratify patients for timing of advanced therapies (transplantation, mechanical support). Patients with peak oxygen consumption $<10\,ml/kg/min$ despite intensification of medical therapy usually benefit from early transplantation, while those with higher levels of oxygen consumption usually benefit most from continued medical therapy and continued close clinical follow-up. Combining the peak oxygen consumption with an index of ventilatory response to exercise, the V_E/V_{CO2} slope (≥ 45 considered abnormal), adds further precision to this assessment process. Conversely, patients with peak oxygen consumption $>20\,ml/kg/min$ and V_E/V_{CO2} slope ≤ 29.9 are at low risk for adverse events.

- Among patients with otherwise unexplained dyspnea following a standard clinical evaluation, CPX can be used as a tool to differentiate between cardiovascular and pulmonary limitations to effort based on the physiological response of the cardiac and pulmonary systems to exercise.
- Other indications for CPX include the assessment of patients with mitochondrial myopathies, development of the exercise prescription in patients with cardiovascular disease or stroke, and the assessment of disability in patients with cardiac or pulmonary disease.

Summary

- Selection of the proper mode of stress testing is highly dependent upon the patient characteristics that are known prior to requesting a stress test.
- It is important to have determined the goal of the stress test in advance in order to gain the desired clinical information.
- Application of Bayes' theorem and consideration of the sensitivity and specificity of the test is important to properly interpret the results of the stress test.
- Exercise is the preferred method of stress because of the important diagnostic and prognostic information obtained from the ECG and hemodynamic responses to exercise.
- The standard exercise ECG stress test should be selected as the first-line test to assess for myocardial ischemia when it is determined that the patient can perform an adequate exercise bout and when the resting ECG is normal or near-normal and the patient is not receiving digitalis.
- Myocardial imaging techniques enhance the diagnostic accuracy of an exercise ECG test and should be used when resting ECG abnormalities that affect repolarization or digitalis therapy is present or a diminished workload is anticipated.

Myocardial imaging also should be used when the indication for the stress test includes localization of myocardial ischemia or myocardial viability. Among patients with intermediate-risk DTS, myocardial imaging provides enhanced risk stratification.

- Selection of a specific myocardial imaging technique should depend upon patient-related characteristics, the type of stress modality requested, and local availability and expertise. Use of myocardial imaging adds time to the stress session, increases costs, and, in the case of MPI, exposes the patient to ionizing radiation.
- Pharmacological stress testing is indicated in situations where the patient cannot perform an adequate exercise ECG test. When pharmacological agents are used, concomitant myocardial imaging is required because of the lower incidence of ST-segment alterations and the associated nonspecific nature of induced chest pain.
- CPX has established use in the HF population and with unexplained dyspnea. Indications for CPX are expected to expand.
- An algorithm for selecting the proper mode of stress testing for the individual patient with suspected or known ischemic heart disease is presented in Figure 11.2.

References

Balady, G.J., Arena, R., Sietsema, K. et al., American Heart Association Exercise, Cardiac Rehabilitation, and Prevention committee of the Council on Clinical Cardiology; Council on Epidemiology and Prevention; Council on Peripheral Vascular Disease; Interdisciplinary Council on Quality of Care and Outcomes Research (2010). Clinician's Guide to cardiopulmonary exercise testing in adults: a scientific statement from the American Heart Association. *Circulation* 122: 191–225.

Bouzas-Mosquera, A., Peteiro, J., Alvarez-García, N. et al. (2009). Prognostic value of exercise echocardiography in patients with left bundle branch block. *JACC Cardiovasc. Imaging* 2: 251–259.

Cheng, V.Y., Berman, D.S., Rozanski, A. et al. (2011). Performance of the traditional age, sex, and angina typicality-based approach for estimating pretest probability of angiographically significant coronary artery disease in patients undergoing coronary computed tomographic angiography: results from the multinational coronary CT angiography evaluation for clinical outcomes: an international multicenter registry (CONFIRM). *Circulation* 124: 2423–2432.

Diamond, G.A. and Forrester, J.S. (1979). Analysis of probability as an aid in the clinical diagnosis of coronary-artery disease. *N. Engl. J. Med.* 300: 1350–1358.

Douglas, P.S., Garcia, M.J., Haines, D.E. et al. (2011). ACCF/ASE/AHA/ASNC/HFSA/HRS/SCAI/SCCM/SCCT/SCMR 2011 appropriate use criteria for echocardiography. *J. Am. Soc. Echocardiogr.* 24: 234.

Fihn, S.D., Gardin, J.M., Abrams, J. et al. (2012). ACCF/AHA/ACP/AATS/PCNA/SCAI/STS guideline for the diagnosis and management of patients with stable ischemic heart disease: executive summary: a report of the American College of Cardiology Foundation/American Heart Association task force on practice guidelines, and the American College of Physicians, American Association for Thoracic Surgery, Preventive Cardiovascular Nurses Association, Society for Cardiovascular Angiography and Interventions, and Society of Thoracic Surgeons. *J. Am. Coll. Cardiol.* 60: 2564–2603.

Geleijnse, M.L., Vigna, C., Kasprzak, J.D. et al. (2000). Usefulness and limitations of dobutamine-atropine stress echocardiography for the diagnosis of coronary artery disease in patients with left bundle branch block. A multicentre study. *Eur. Heart J.* 21: 1666–1773.

Henzlova, M.J., Duvall, W.L., Einstein, A.J. et al. (2016). ASNC imaging guidelines for SPECT nuclear cardiology procedures: stress, protocols, and tracers. *J. Nucl. Cardiol.* 23: 606–639.

Hlatky, M.A., Boineau, R.E., Higginbotham, M.B. et al. (1989). A brief self-administered questionnaire to determine functional capacity (the Duke Activity Status Index). *Am. J. Cardiol.* 64: 651–654.

Patterson, R.E. and Horowitz, S.F. (1989). Importance of epidemiology and biostatistics in deciding clinical strategies for using diagnostic tests: a simplified approach using examples from coronary artery disease. *J. Am. Coll. Cardiol.* 13: 1653–1665.

Pryor, D.B., Shaw, L., McCants, C.B. et al. (1993). Value of the history and physical in identifying patients at increased risk for coronary artery disease. *Ann. Intern. Med.* 118: 81–90.

Wolk, M.J., Bailey, S.R., Doherty, J.U. et al., American College of Cardiology Foundation Appropriate Use Criteria Task Force (2014). ACCF/AHA/ASE/ASNC/HFSA/HRS/SCAI/SCCT/SCMR/STS 2013 multimodality appropriate use criteria for the detection and risk assessment of stable ischemic heart disease: a report of the American College of Cardiology Foundation appropriate use criteria task force, American Heart Association, American Society of Echocardiography, American Society of Nuclear Cardiology, Heart Failure Society of America, Heart Rhythm Society, Society for Cardiovascular Angiography and Interventions, Society of Cardiovascular Computed Tomography, Society for Cardiovascular Magnetic Resonance, and Society of Thoracic Surgeons. *J. Am. Coll. Cardiol.* 63: 380–406.

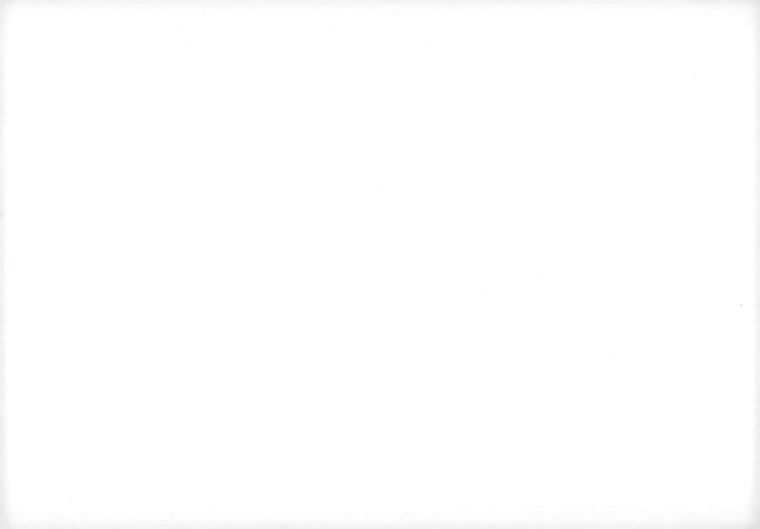

12 Exercise-induced Cardiac Arrhythmias

Bryon A. Gentile

Introduction

Exercise can provoke or suppress cardiac arrhythmias in both healthy patients and those with underlying heart disease. Considerable debate exists regarding the clinical significance of ventricular arrhythmias that occur during exercise, particularly ventricular premature contractions (VPCs). In general, VPCs should raise concern among patients with a history of cardiomyopathy, valvular heart disease, or myocardial ischemia, and patients with a family history of sudden death.

Supraventricular arrhythmias induced by exercise, such as atrial tachycardia (AT) or atrial fibrillation (AF), are uncommon, while atrioventricular (AV) conduction time is often altered by exercise. Interventricular blocks tend to be rate-dependent, and the development of a rate-related left bundle branch block (LBBB) during exercise precludes assessment for ischemia. Exercise may provoke or suppress pre-excitation in patients with Wolff-Parkinson-White (WPW) pattern/syndrome and ST-segment abnormalities are common. As a result, the ECG is often non-diagnostic for ischemia.

Pocket Guide to Stress Testing, Second Edition. Edited by Dennis A. Tighe and Bryon A. Gentile.
© 2020 John Wiley & Sons Ltd. Published 2020 by John Wiley & Sons Ltd.

This chapter reviews current knowledge on electrophysiologic responses of the heart in response to exercise, in conjunction with the classification, diagnosis, and clinical significance of exercise-induced arrhythmias.

Equipment

Appropriate preparations, including proper skin preparation, (Chapter 2) is helpful in minimizing excessive noise and ECG artifact. A multi-lead ECG system is important to identifying exercise-induced arrhythmias, as a single-lead system is insufficient. If a two-lead system is to be employed, it is suggested that a minimum of one inferior lead (II or aVF) be added to modified bipolar lead V5 as this will allow for optimal identification of the P-wave, which can be helpful in distinguishing supraventricular from ventricular arrhythmias, as well as assessing for advanced conduction abnormalities. Our laboratory utilizes a three-lead system (II, V1, and V5) capable of obtaining and storing a full 12-lead ECG on demand and when sustained arrhythmias are noted.

Electrophysiologic Effects of Exercise

Exercise is known to alter events in the myocardium which may lead to the production or inhibition of ectopic impulse formation. In addition, conduction through the AV node may be enhanced or depressed.

Exercise-induced arrhythmias are generated by enhanced sympathetic tone and/or increased myocardial oxygen demand. The increased sympathetic tone may stimulate ectopic Purkinje pacemaker activity by accelerating phase 4 depolarization, provoking spontaneous discharge and leading to increased automaticity.

Local tissue hypoxia is produced when the increased myocardial oxygen demand exceeds oxygen supply and induces a temporal dispersion of depolarization and repolarization in addition to alterations of the cardiac conduction velocity. As a result, myocardial ischemia can provide a substrate for the initiation of ectopic arrhythmias via automatic and re-entrant mechanisms.

Myocardial oxygen supply/demand mismatch can be observed not only during high-level exercise but also in the immediate post-exercise period. Exercise-induced peripheral arteriolar dilation coupled with the reduction in cardiac output (Q), resulting from diminished venous return due to the sudden termination of muscular activity at the end of exercise, may lead to an abrupt drop in BP and coronary perfusion while the heart rate (HR) remains elevated.

Exercise may also suppress arrhythmias present at rest due to overdrive inhibition of ectopic impulse formation by increases in sinoatrial activity due to increased sympathetic stimulation. Thus, exercise-induced sinus tachycardia may inhibit the automaticity of an ectopic focus as rapid stimulation may result in reduced automaticity of the Purkinje tissue.

Value of Exercise Stress Testing in Diagnosing and Managing Arrhythmias

Exercise ECG stress testing can be useful in the diagnosis of exercise-induced arrhythmias in addition to assessing the efficacy of anti-arrhythmic medications.

Although Holter and event monitors are essential in detecting transient and occult arrhythmias that may not be detected on the resting ECG, exercise stress ECG testing can be valuable in detecting exercise-induced arrhythmias. Holter and event monitors are generally worn by patients during routine daily activity and during light exercise. They are rarely worn during near-maximal or maximal exercise and as a result have limited ability to detect arrhythmias under these conditions. Thus, exercise testing can serve as a supplementary tool in the diagnosis of arrhythmias provoked by near-maximal or maximal exercise. The exercise ECG also has significant value in assessing the efficacy of various anti-arrhythmic agents.

Common indications include:

- Assessment of exertional HR response and effects of rate-controlling medications (e.g. non-dihydropyridine calcium channel blockers and beta-blockers) in patients with chronic AF.
- Assessment of anti-arrhythmic drug therapy in patients with exercise-induced arrhythmias (e.g. AF, VPCs, etc.).
- Provocation of catecholaminergic polymorphic ventricular tachycardia (VT). Exercise-testing is the primary test to diagnose this condition. As long-acting, nonselective beta-blockers are an integral component of therapy for most patients with this condition, the exercise test can also be used to assess the efficacy of therapy.

Cardiac Arrhythmias and Termination of Exercise Testing

In general, it is recommended that exercise be terminated if sustained VT or other arrhythmias that interfere with normal maintenance of Q occur, such as Mobitz type II second-degree or third-degree (complete) AV block.

Although the presence of significant (complex) ventricular arrhythmias is considered to be a relative contraindication to the exercise ECG by some investigators, our laboratory's policy is that exercise ECG testing is not contraindicated when a patient's condition is stable and relatively benign ventricular arrhythmias (e.g. VPCs) are present on the resting ECG. If a complex ventricular rhythm disorder develops during stress testing, exercise should be terminated immediately.

Exercise may be continued when the patient develops benign supraventricular arrhythmias such as atrial premature contraction (APCs), atrial grouped beats, or short runs of AT. Exercise should be stopped if AF or atrial flutter with rapid ventricular response is provoked by exercise.

Classification, Diagnosis, and Clinical Significance of Exercise-Induced Arrhythmias

Arrhythmias may be provoked or suppressed during exercise. Conduction disturbances, including bundle branch blocks, fascicular blocks, and AV block, can also be observed. This section will review common arrhythmias and conduction disturbances encountered during exercise ECG testing.

Sinus Arrhythmias

- Progressive acceleration of the sinus rate is expected during multistage exercise ECG testing. Predicted maximal HR typically varies by age. In our laboratory we estimate the age-predicted maximal HR using the formula (220 bpm – age).
- When the expected increment of the sinus rate is not observed during exercise ECG testing in patients not taking AV nodal blocking agents, dysfunction of the sinus node (e.g. sick sinus syndrome) may be present.
- Sinus arrhythmia and wandering atrial pacemaker are quite common in the immediate post-exercise period. These presence of these alone are not typically associated with pathology.

Atrial Arrhythmias

- Exercise-induced APCs and atrial grouped beats (Figures 12.1 and 12.2) are common in normal and diseased hearts. Differentiation between APCs with aberrant ventricular conduction and VPCs can be challenging. The concept of the full compensatory pause in VPCs and non-full-compensatory pause in APCs cannot be applied readily during very rapid HRs because the coupling interval in both situations approaches the R-R interval of the

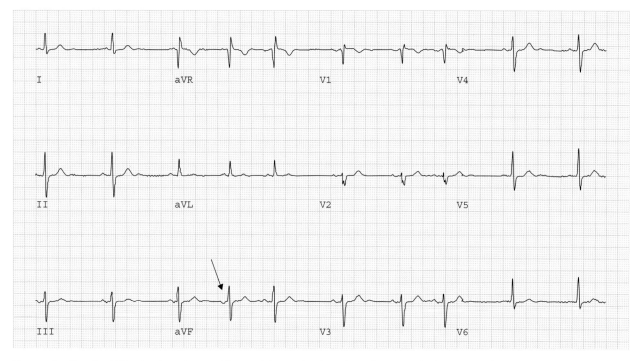

Figure 12.1 Baseline ECG taken in a 68-year-old man with sinus bradycardia with sinus arrhythmia. A single APC is noted (arrow).

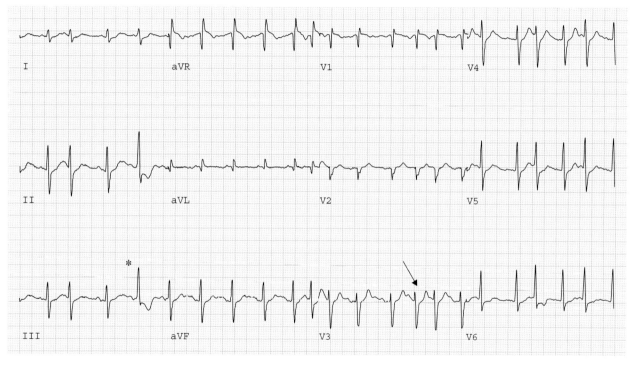

Figure 12.2 Exercise ECG in the same 68-year-old man. Note an atrial premature contraction (APC) with aberrant ventricular conduction (asterisk) and grouped atrial couplets (arrow).

basic rhythm. Frequent occurrence of ventricular fusion beats with VPCs make them more difficult to distinguish from APCs with aberrant ventricular conduction.

- Sustained paroxysmal AT induced by exercise is rare. Short episodes of AT induced by exercise are not uncommon (Figure 12.2).
- AF or flutter induced by exercise is uncommon, occurring in less than 1% of individuals undergoing exercise ECG stress testing (Figures 12.3 and 12.4). While these exercise-induced arrhythmias can occur in healthy patients, they can also be seen in patients with rheumatic heart disease, hyperthyroidism, WPW syndrome, and cardiomyopathies.

AV Junctional Arrhythmias

- The incidence of exercise-induced junctional premature contractions (JPCs) is uncertain as most investigators do not distinguish between APCs and JPCs. In addition, it can be difficult or impossible to distinguish between these two arrhythmias during exercise at rapid HRs.
- Similarly, the incidence of exercise-induced junctional tachycardia is unknown as these are generally grouped under "SVT" and can be difficult to distinguish from paroxysmal AT.
- The clinical significance of JPCs and paroxysmal junctional tachycardia is not known, but probably is similar to that of APCs and AT. The presence of junctional tachycardia alone is not indicative of ischemia.
- A transient episode of junctional escape rhythm, with or without wandering atrial pacemaker, is not uncommon during the recovery period.

Ventricular Arrhythmias

Ventricular arrhythmias, particularly VPCs, may be induced or abolished by exercise in normal subjects as well as in patients with structural heart disease, including those with coronary artery disease (CAD). Considerable debate exists among investigators regarding the clinical significance of VPCs. In general, the presence of VPCs at rest should

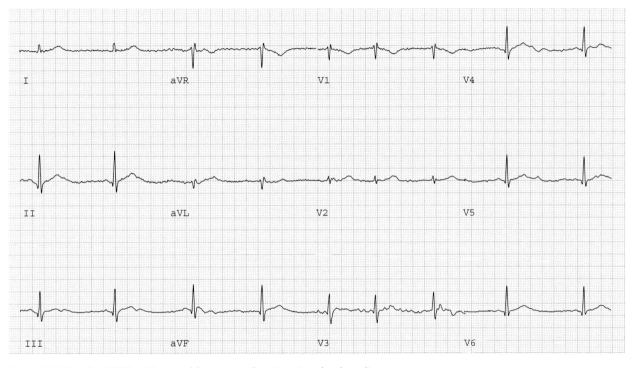

Figure 12.3 Baseline ECG in a 72-year-old woman with resting sinus bradycardia.

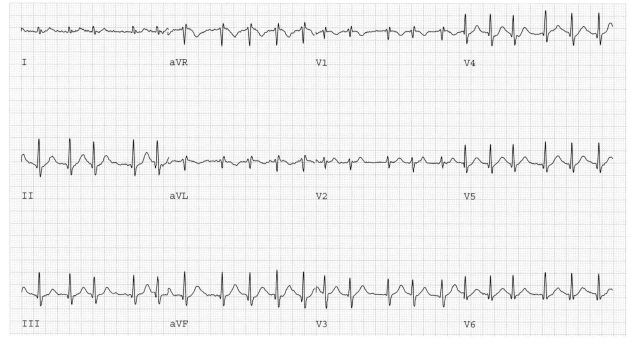

Figure 12.4 Exercise ECG in the same 72-year-old woman who developed AF during exercise. The patient spontaneously converted back to sinus rhythm in late recovery. Echocardiography demonstrated no structural heart disease.

raise concern in patients with a history of cardiomyopathy, valvular heart disease, myocardial ischemia, and among patients with a family history of sudden death. Consideration should be given to:

- Site of the origin of VPCs (right vs left ventricle)
- VPCs at rest
- VPCs induced by exercise (onset of VPCs in relation to the amount of exercise)
- VPCs abolished by exercise
- Unifocal vs multifocal VPCs
- Grouped vs isolated VPCs
- Relation to the development of VT/VF
- Relation to the presence or absence of CAD
- Relation to the risk of developing future coronary event

Isolated, unifocal VPCs are the most common arrhythmia encountered during exercise testing. Multifocal VPCs and grouped (three or more) VPCs or VT are more common in patients with CAD (Figures 12.5 and 12.6).

Diagnosis of Ventricular Arrhythmias

- Differentiating VT from SVT with aberrant conduction or pre-existing bundle branch block can be challenging.
- Similarly, supraventricular tachyarrhythmias, particularly AF in the setting of WPW syndrome, closely mimics VT or even VF (Figures 12.7 and 12.8).
- Multifocal VPCs may be diagnosed erroneously when frequent ventricular fusion beats in unifocal VPCs are seen during rapid HR induced by exercise.
- In addition, APCs or JPCs with aberrant ventricular conduction can mimic VPCs.

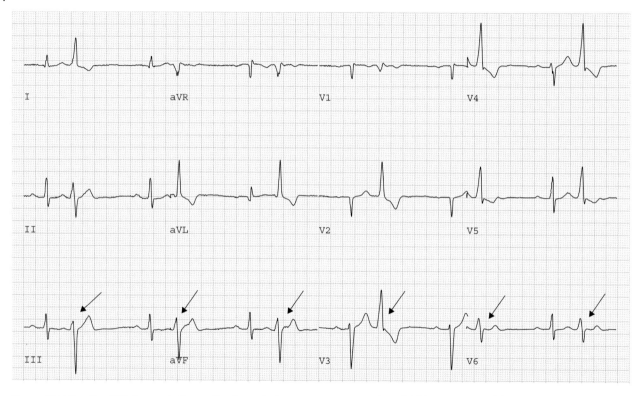

Figure 12.5 Baseline ECG demonstrating unifocal ventricular premature contractions (VPCs) in a 75-year-old man with known CAD undergoing exercise testing for evaluation of a chest pain syndrome. Note that the frequent VPCs occur in a pattern of bigeminy (arrows).

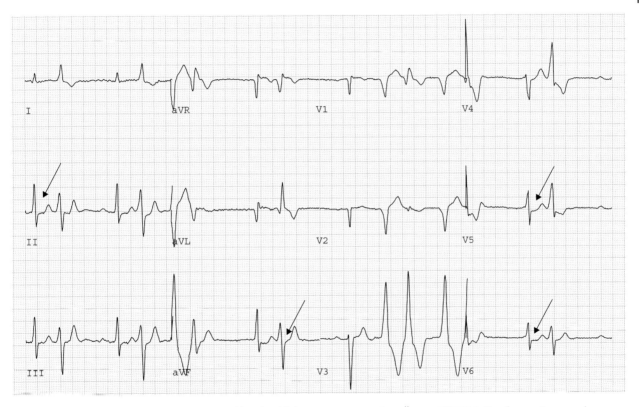

Figure 12.6 Recovery ECG in the same 75-year-old male with known coronary artery disease demonstrating frequent grouped ventricular premature contractions (VPCs). Note the associated ST-segment depression in inferolateral leads indicative of ischemia (arrows). At coronary angiography, the patient was found to have severe, three-vessel CAD.

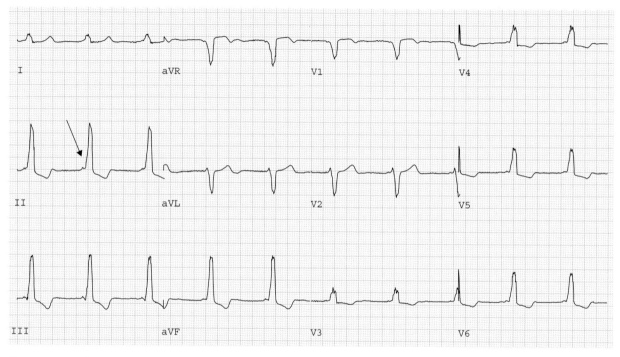

Figure 12.7 Baseline ECG in a 32-year-old woman with WPW syndrome. Note the short PR interval and delta wave (arrow).

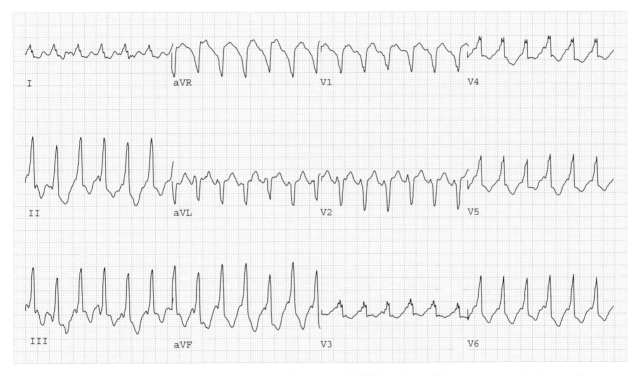

Figure 12.8 Peak exercise ECG racing in the same 32-year-old woman with WPW syndrome. This wide complex rhythm can often mimic ventricular tachycardia (VT). Note that the QRS morphology and axis are identical to the baseline, making VT unlikely.

- The aforementioned differential diagnosis can be challenging; however, it is important to distinguish these arrhythmias due to their differing clinical significance.

Ventricular Arrhythmias Induced by Exercise

As previously noted, VPCs are commonly encountered during exercise and are concerning in patients with a history of cardiomyopathy, valvular heart disease, ischemia or family history of sudden cardiac death. Some studies suggest that frequent ventricular ectopy (defined as the presence of seven or more VPCs per minute, ventricular bigeminy or trigeminy, ventricular couplets or triplets, VT, ventricular flutter, torsade de pointes, or ventricular fibrillation), particularly when it occurs during the recovery period, is an independent predictor of mortality.

- VPCs triggered at low levels of exercise are commonly associated with CAD, particularly if multifocal in origin and associated with concomitant ST-segment deviations (Figures 12.5 and 12.6)
- Exercise-induced VT is highly suggestive of underlying heart disease. Most commonly it is associated with CAD, however it can also occur in patients with an underlying cardiomyopathy. Alternatively, exercise can induce catecholamine-triggered polymorphic VT or VT from the right ventricular outflow tract (Figures 12.9 and 12.10).

Exercise-Induced Ventricular Fibrillation

Although typically associated with CAD-induced ischemia or in patients with hypertrophic cardiomyopathy and LV outflow tract obstruction, ventricular fibrillation can also occur unpredictably during strenuous exercise. Fortunately, exercise-induced ventricular fibrillation is rarely encountered.

Conclusions

- VPCs are the most commonly encountered ventricular arrhythmia noted during exercise. VPCs are often suppressed with exercise as the sinus rate accelerates.

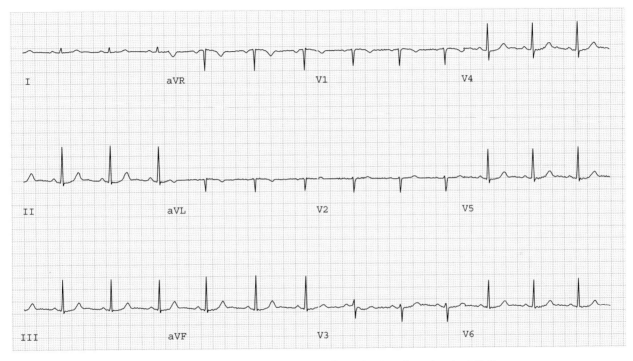

Figure 12.9 Baseline ECG in a 54-year-old woman undergoing an ETT for evaluation of exertional palpitations.

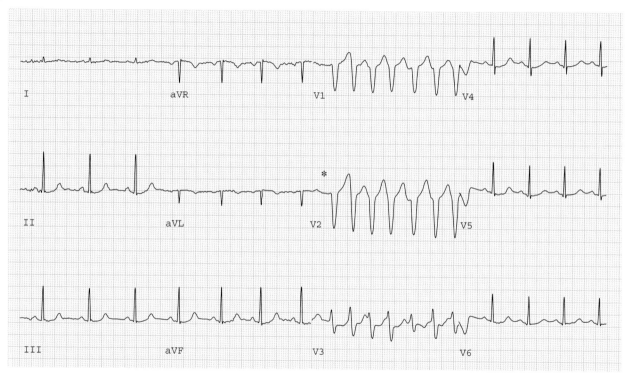

Figure 12.10 Exercise ECG in the same 54-year-old woman demonstrating non-sustained ventricular tachycardia (VT) (asterisk). Note the left bundle branch morphology and absence of ST-segment alterations and QRS transition after lead V2. Echocardiography demonstrated a structurally normal heart. EP study confirmed the right ventricular outflow tract as the origin of the VT, which was successfully ablated.

- Multifocal VPCs may be encountered in healthy patients as well as those with structural heart disease.
- Exercise-induced ventricular arrhythmias are more common in patients with underlying heart disease.
- Ventricular arrhythmias induced at low levels of exercise are suggestive of the presence of CAD.
- Exercise-induced VPCs or VT in the absence of ST-segment alterations is not necessarily indicative of underlying CAD. Exercise-induced VT may the result of an underlying cardiomyopathy, catecholamine-triggered event, or originate from the right ventricular outflow tract.
- Some studies suggest that frequent ventricular ectopy, particularly in the recovery period, is an independent predictor of mortality.

AV Conduction Abnormalities

It is not uncommon to observe alterations in the PR-interval during and/or immediately after exercise. Shortening of the PR-interval is benign and likely the result of increased sympathetic tone; it occurs commonly among young healthy individuals.

First-Degree AV Block

- First-degree AV block is occasionally observed in the exercise laboratory during the late portion of the exercise or immediately after the exercise period. This phenomenon is likely related to increased vagal tone. It may also be encountered in conditions or with medications that prolong AV conduction time (e.g. myocardial inflammation, digitalis, beta-blockers, non-dihydropyridine calcium channel blockers).
- Some patients may develop Mobitz type I (Wenckebach) second-degree AV block following first-degree AV block.
- First-degree AV block in the absence of ST-segmentation alterations is not indicative of CAD.

Second-Degree AV Block

- The development of Mobitz type I (Wenckebach) second-degree AV block is occasionally encountered during exercise testing and is probably the result of increased vagal tone. Therefore, exercise-induced Mobitz type I second-degree AV block may be physiologic in nature.
- Mobitz type II second-degree AV block is uncommon and may be a rate-related phenomenon that appears as the sinus rate is accelerated beyond a critical level. It may also be encountered in patients with CAD or aortic stenosis and may be a harbinger of complete heart block (Figures 12.11 and 12.12).

Complete AV Block

- Complete (third-degree) AV block is a relative contraindication to exercise ECG testing due to the risk of ventricular arrhythmias.
- Exercise testing can be performed in patients with congenital complete AV block in the absence of coexisting congenital anomalies precluding safe exercise to assess the HR response to stress.
- Complete heart block induced by exercise is uncommon, but may be the result of AV nodal ischemia.
- If complete heart block develops during exercise testing, exercise should be terminated.

Intraventricular Blocks

- Intraventricular blocks may be observed during exercise ECG testing and are primarily a rate-related phenomenon. Indeed, right bundle branch block (RBBB) or LBBB occurs during exercise as the sinus rate increases beyond the individual's critical rate as a result of concealed bundle branch block (Figures 12.13–12.15).
- Exercise may also induce left anterior, left posterior, or bifascicular blocks.

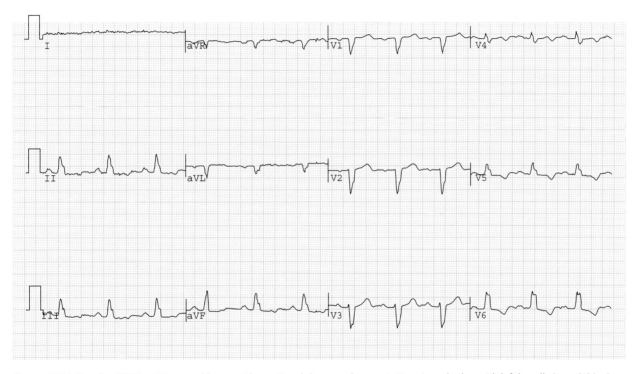

Figure 12.11 Baseline ECG in a 78-year-old man with exertional dyspnea demonstrating sinus rhythm with left bundle branch block (LBBB).

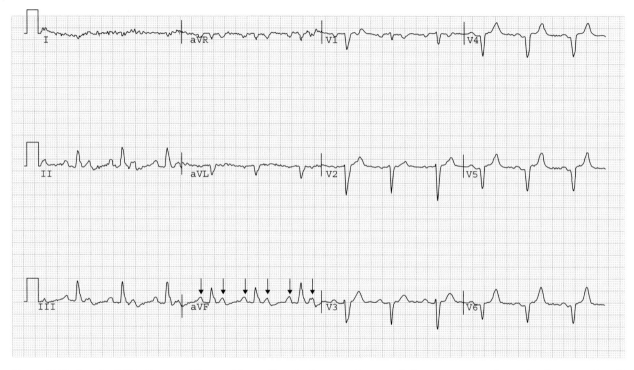

Figure 12.12 Exercise ECG in the same 78-year-old man. Note the inappropriate ventricular rate response due to development of 2:1 AV block. P waves (arrows) are often best discerned in inferior leads. A permanent pacemaker was placed with resolution of dyspnea.

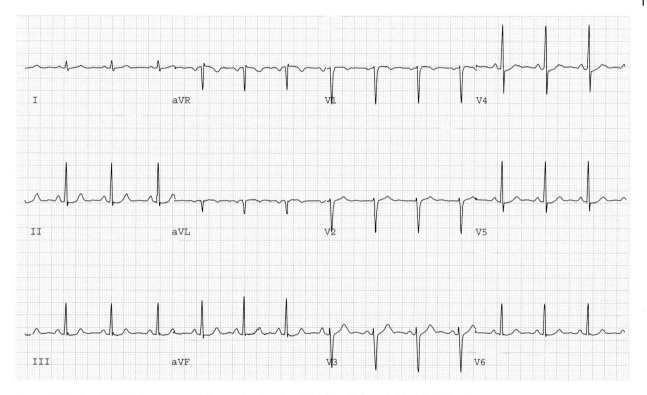

Figure 12.13 Baseline ECG in a 62 year-old man who developed left bundle branch block (LBBB) with exercise.

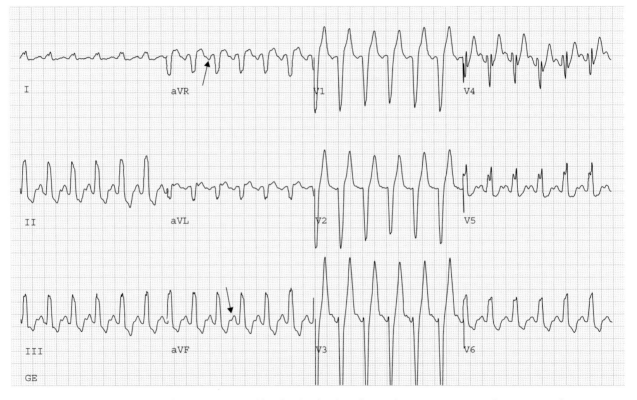

Figure 12.14 Peak exercise ECG in the same 61-year-old male who developed LBBB during exercise. Note the presence of sinus p-waves (arrows) with a 1:1 relationship to the QRS complexes, excluding exercise-induced ventricular tachycardia.

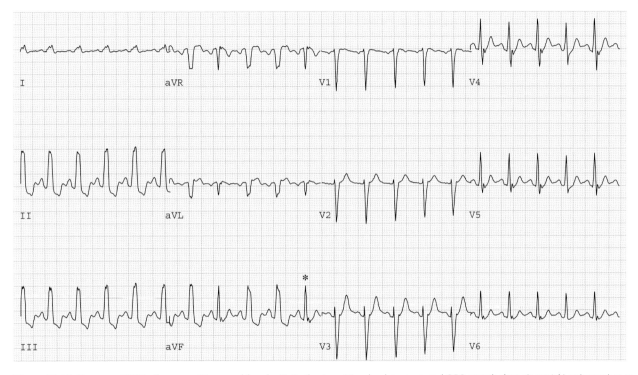

Figure 12.15 Recovery ECG in the same 61-year-old male. Note the transition back to a normal QRS morphology (asterisk) at lower heart rates.

- The development of an intraventricular block during exercise is not diagnostic for CAD. In one study, development of an exercise-induced LBBB independently predicted death and major cardiovascular events.
- While the development of an exercise-induced LBBB precludes interpretation of the exercise ECG, development of an exercise-induced RBBB does not.

Tachycardia-Bradycardia Syndrome

Tachycardia-bradycardia syndrome is a complication of sick-sinus-syndrome characterized by alternating tachycardia and bradycardia. It is typically observed in older patients and those with organic heart disease.

WPW Syndrome

- Exercise may provoke, suppress, or have no effect on pre-excitation in patients with WPW pattern/syndrome.
- Significant ST-segment depression may be observed in patients with WPW undergoing exercise testing, particularly when pre-excitation remains unsuppressed with exercise. As a result, ST-segment changes in patients with WPW are non-diagnostic for ischemia (Figures 12.16 and 12.17).
- The prevalence of exercise-induced tachyarrhythmias is low in patients with WPW syndrome.
- Suppression of pre-excitation with exercise can identify patients at lower risk of sudden death.

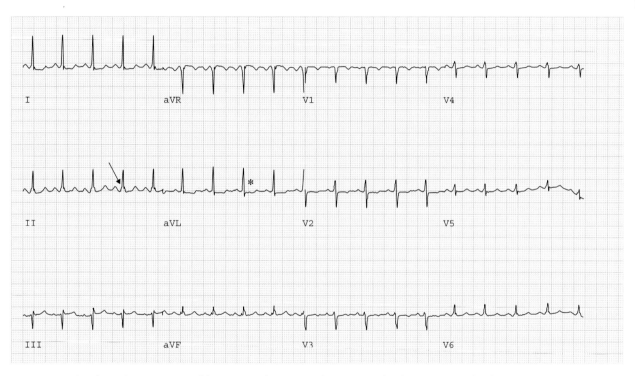

Figure 12.16 Baseline ECG in a 26 year-old-woman with WPW syndrome. Note the short PR-interval, delta wave (arrow), and non-specific ST-segment abnormalities (asterisk).

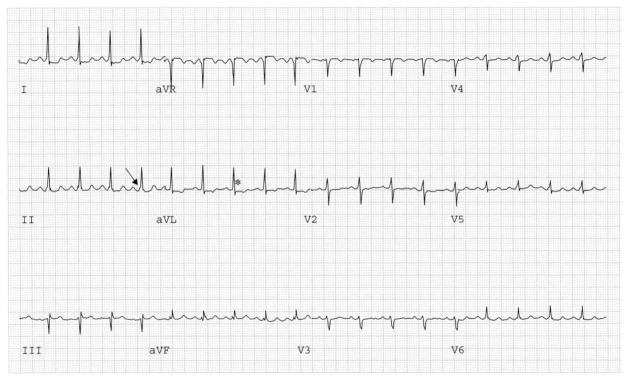

Figure 12.17 Recovery ECG in the same 26 year-old-woman. Note the persistent ST-T abnormalities (asterisk) and delta wave (arrow).

Summary

- Exercise is capable of provoking or suppressing arrhythmias.
- Ventricular arrhythmias are the primary concern in the exercise laboratory.
- VPCs are the most common exercise-induced arrhythmia, but may commonly be suppressed with exercise.
- VPCs should raise concern in patients with a history of cardiomyopathy, valvular heart disease, myocardial ischemia, and among patients with a family history of sudden death.
- In general, exercise-induced ventricular arrhythmias are more common in patients with CAD or structural heart disease than in healthy individuals.
- CAD should be suspected when ventricular arrhythmias are provoked at low levels of exercise.
- Exercise-induced VPCs or VT with ST-segment changes is strongly suggestive of underlying CAD. Exercise-induced VT in the absence of ST-segment changes may the result of an underlying cardiomyopathy, be catecholamine-triggered, or originate from the right ventricular outflow tract.
- Exercise may induce first-degree AV block or Mobitz type I (Wenckebach) second-degree AV block in healthy individuals due to increased vagal tone. It may also be encountered in conditions or with medications that prolong AV conduction time (e.g. myocardial inflammation, digitalis, beta-blockers, non-dihydropyridine calcium channel blockers).
- The occurrence of exercise-induced bundle branch block or fascicular block is a rate-dependent phenomenon and is not indicative of CAD.
- The prevalence of exercise-induced tachyarrhythmias is low in patients with WPW pattern/syndrome.

References

Aleong, R.G., Singh, S.M., Levinson, J.R., and Milan, D.J. (2009). Catecholamine challenge unmasking high-risk features in the Wolff-Parkinson-White syndrome. *Europace* 11: 1396–1398.

Atwood, J.E., Myers, J., Sullivan, M. et al. (1988). Maximal exercise testing and gas exchange in patients with chronic atrial fibrillation. *J. Am. Coll. Cardiol.* 11: 508–513.

Beckerman, J., Mathur, A., Stahr, S. et al. (2005). Exercise-induced ventricular arrhythmias and cardiovascular death. *Ann. Noninvasive Electrocardiol.* 10: 47–52.

Dewey, F.E., Kapoor, J.R., Williams, R.S. et al. (2008). Ventricular arrhythmias during clinical treadmill testing and prognosis. *Arch. Intern. Med.* 168: 225–234.

Fletcher, G.F., Ades, P.A., Kligfield, P. et al., on behalf of the American Heart Association Exercise, Cardiac Rehabilitation, and Prevention Committee of the Council on Clinical Cardiology, Council on Nutrition, Physical Activity and Metabolism, Council on Cardiovascular and Stroke Nursing, and Council on Epidemiology and Prevention (2013). Exercise standards for testing and training: a scientific statement from the American Heart Association. *Circulation* 128: 873–934.

Frolkis, J.P., Pothier, C.E., Blackstone, E.H., and Lauer, M.S. (2003). Frequent ventricular ectopy after exercise as a predictor of death. *N. Engl. J. Med.* 348: 781–790. Erratum in: N. Engl. J. Med. 2003; 348: 1508.

Grady, T.A., Chiu, A.C., Snader, C.E. et al. (1998). Prognostic significance of exercise-induced left bundle-branch block. *JAMA* 279: 153–156.

Jezior, M.R., Kent, S.M., and Atwood, J.E. (2005). Exercise testing in Wolff-Parkinson-White syndrome: case report with ECG and literature review. *Chest* 127: 1454–1457.

Peller, O.G., Moses, J.W., and Kligfield, P. (1988). Exercise-induced atrioventricular block: report of three cases. *Am. Heart J.* 115: 1315–1317.

Yuzuki, Y., Horie, M., Makita, T. et al. (1997). Exercise-induced second-degree atrioventricular block. *Jpn. Circ. J.* 61: 268–271.

13 Complications

Bryon A. Gentile

Introduction

The exercise ECG test is designed to obtain diagnostic and functional data regarding the cardiovascular system. As a result, it is not without inherent risk and complications such as sudden death, acute myocardial infarction (MI), and ventricular arrhythmias can and do occur.

The incidence of various complications is influenced by many factors, such as the method of exercise and patient co-morbidities. Fortunately, the incidence of serious (life-threatening) complications is rather low and generally quoted at about 1:10 000.

A survey study from the VA healthcare system with over 60 000 exercise-based tests performed, reported a major complication rate of 1.2 per 10 000 tests with no deaths reported.

Complications of exercise ECG stress testing are listed in Table 13.1.

Pocket Guide to Stress Testing, Second Edition. Edited by Dennis A. Tighe and Bryon A. Gentile.
© 2020 John Wiley & Sons Ltd. Published 2020 by John Wiley & Sons Ltd.

Table 13.1 Complications of exercise ECG stress testing.

Cardiac complications
Arrhythmias
Tachyarrhythmias
Atrial fibrillation
Supraventricular tachycardia
Junctional tachycardia
Ventricular tachycardia
Ventricular fibrillation
Bradyarrhythmias
Sinus bradycardia
Junctional bradycardia
AV block
Ventricular escape rhythms
Asystole
Angina pectoris
Myocardial infarction
Congestive heart failure
Hypertension
Hypotension and shock
Sudden death
Syncope
Non-cardiac complications
Injuries related to falls
Claudication
Cerebrovascular accident
Ill-defined and miscellaneous complications
Severe fatigue, dizziness, malaise, myalgias, arthralgias

Cardiac Complications

Arrhythmias

Tachyarrhythmias

Cardiac arrhythmias are the most common complication of exercise ECG testing. Premature atrial and ventricular contractions (APCs and VPCs) are common in healthy individuals. The VPC burden typically improves as heart rate (HR) increases with exercise. Ventricular ectopy is concerning in patients with a cardiomyopathy, valvular heart disease, myocardial ischemia, or a family history of sudden death. Complex ventricular ectopy that occurs at a low workload or with an ischemic ECG response is a marker of increased risk. Some studies have suggested that ventricular ectopy in the recovery period can be an independent predictor of death.

Ventricular tachycardia (VT) and ventricular fibrillation (VF) are rare events that can lead to sudden death. Unsustained VT during exercise may simply be a marker of underlying heart disease; prognosis is associated more strongly with the severity of the underlying cardiac disease. Polymorphic VT and VF are highly suggestive of myocardial ischemia and underlying coronary artery disease (CAD). Monomorphic VT can be triggered by multifocal VPCs, the R-on-T phenomenon, and grouped VPCs.

Bradyarrhythmias

Various bradyarrhythmias are uncommon but can occur during and after exercise. The most common bradyarrhythmia experienced prior to beginning exercise is sinus bradycardia, which is often the result of treatment with beta-blockers and non-dihydropyridine calcium channel blockers. Blunted HR response during exercise is often the result of these medications. In the absence of these medications, sick sinus syndrome should be suspected when the HR response to exercise is inadequate.

Sudden Death

The most feared complication of exercise testing is sudden death, which is typically associated with VT or VF. Predictors of sudden death during testing include hypotensive and blunted BP responses to exercise. A subgroup at increased risk for exercise-induced sudden death is the high-risk subgroup with proven CAD associated with exercise-induced hypotension.

The chance of sudden death may increase during or immediately after exercise in patients undergoing exercise testing following an acute coronary syndrome (ACS), particularly when significant ST-segment depression, angina, or hypotension is provoked. As a result, healthcare professionals must be aware of these findings and alter testing as appropriate.

Angina Pectoris and MI

The risk of provoking a MI in patients undergoing exercise testing is low. The risk increases among patients with known multi-vessel CAD as well those undergoing exercise testing following ACS.

The development of angina pectoris is more common than that of MI due to the supply and demand mismatch imposed by stenotic coronary arteries. Healthcare professionals supervising exercise testing must be aware of such symptoms and monitor for concurrent ST segment changes, arrhythmia, and abnormal BP responses. Oftentimes, ECG abnormalities may precede symptoms of angina. The ischemic cascade suggests that regional systolic dysfunction may precede both ECG abnormalities and the clinical symptom of angina.

Congestive Heart Failure

The core concept of exercise testing for the diagnosis of obstructive CAD is to provoke the supply/demand mismatch leading to objective evidence of myocardial ischemia. The ischemic cascade suggests the development of early diastolic dysfunction prior to the development of systolic dysfunction, ECG abnormalities, and symptoms of angina. As a result, there is an increase in left atrial and subsequently pulmonary venous pressure which can lead to symptoms of congestive heart failure (CHF). These symptoms may include exercise-induced coughing and dyspnea.

Hypertension and Hypotension

An increase in SBP is a normal physiologic response to exercise (average rise in SBP is about 10 mmHg/MET). An exaggerated SBP response to exercise, defined by some as ≥210 mmHg for men and ≥190 mmHg for women, may predict future development of systemic hypertension and possibly other adverse cardiovascular events.

The occurrence of hypotension or a blunted BP response to progressive exercise represents a significant concern as it is usually observed among patients with advanced multi-vessel CAD, aortic outflow obstruction, and/or left ventricular (LV) dysfunction. This response can be complicated by ventricular arrhythmias and can be particularly true among patients who have suffered a recent MI.

Noncardiac Complications

Musculoskeletal Trauma

Injuries related to falls can be observed during exercise testing, particularly in patients with gait instability. The healthcare professional supervising exercise testing should monitor for worsening gait instability and terminate exercise if patients cannot continue to exercise safely.

Claudication

Atherosclerosis is a systemic disease and can manifest in the vasculature of the lower extremities. With exercise the same supply/demand mismatch occurring in the myocardium can occur in the musculature of the lower extremities, resulting in claudication. The major consequence of this during exercise is that testing end prematurely due to limiting claudication.

Cerebrovascular Accidents

Cerebrovascular accidents connected with exercise testing have been reported but the relationship to exercise has not been clearly defined. We are not aware of a patient at our institution that has suffered a cerebrovascular accident as a result of exercise ECG stress testing. Known significant cerebrovascular disease is a relative contraindication for vasodilator stress testing.

Ill-Defined and Miscellaneous Complications

There are other ill-defined complications that may potentially occur in connection with exercise testing. These may include severe fatigue, dizziness, near syncope or syncope, general malaise, myalgias, or arthralgias. Symptoms must be evaluated carefully by the healthcare professional supervising the exercise test.

Summary
• Serious complications resulting from exercise ECG stress testing are rare, and generally reported to occur in about 1 in 10 000 tests. • To minimize the risk of complications, the objectives of every test as well as potential contraindications should be evaluated prior to exercise testing. • Patients with advanced CAD or those having suffered a recent ACS are at highest risk of complications. • The most serious complications include severe angina, exercise-induced hypotension, ventricular arrhythmias, acute MI, or even cardiac death. • Complications may be prevented or minimized when the patient is properly selected and exercise testing is properly performed and supervised.

References

Beckerman, J., Mathur, A., Stahr, S. et al. (2005). Exercise-induced ventricular arrhythmias and cardiovascular death. *Ann. Noninvasive Electrocardiol.* 10: 47–52.

Bruce, R.A., Hossack, K.F., DeRouuen, T.A., and Hofer, V. (1983). Enhanced risk assessment for primary coronary heart disease events by maximal exercise testing: 10 years' experience of Seattle Heart Watch. *J. Am. Coll. Cardiol.* 2: 565–573.

Dewey, F.E., Kapoor, J.R., Williams, R.S. et al. (2008). Ventricular arrhythmias during clinical treadmill testing and prognosis. *Arch. Intern. Med.* 168: 225–234.

Fletcher, G.F., Ades, P.A., Kligfield, P. et al., on behalf of the American Heart Association Exercise, Cardiac Rehabilitation, and Prevention Committee of the Council on Clinical Cardiology, Council on Nutrition, Physical Activity and Metabolism, Council on Cardiovascular and Stroke Nursing, and Council on Epidemiology and Prevention (2013). Exercise standards for testing and training: a scientific statement from the American Heart Association. *Circulation* 128: 873–934.

Myers, J., Voodi, L., Umann, T., and Froelicher, V.F. (2000). A survey of exercise testing: methods, utilization, interpretation, and safety in the VAHCS. *J. Cardpulm. Rehabil.* 20: 251–258.

Nesto, R.W. and Kowalchuk, G.J. (1987). The ischemic cascade: temporal sequence of hemodynamic, electrocardiographic and symptomatic expressions of ischemia. *Am. J. Cardiol.* 57: 23C–30C.

14 Interpretation

Bryon A. Gentile and Dennis A. Tighe

Introduction

There are numerous physiologic responses to exercise, including ECG changes, that are to be expected in normal individuals during exercise. It is essential to understand expected changes to accurately interpret changes suggestive of myocardial ischemia.

In general, there are three major ischemic responses that may occur during an exercise ECG test:

- Electrical events: ECG changes: ST-segment deviations and various arrhythmias.
- Hemodynamic events: alterations in blood pressure (BP) and heart rate (HR).
- Symptomatic manifestations: such as chest pain and dyspnea.

Among these ischemic responses, electrical events, such as ST-segment depression, are the traditional criteria for the diagnosis of coronary artery disease (CAD). As with any test, there are numerous factors that may influence the results (Table 14.1).

Pocket Guide to Stress Testing, Second Edition. Edited by Dennis A. Tighe and Bryon A. Gentile.
© 2020 John Wiley & Sons Ltd. Published 2020 by John Wiley & Sons Ltd.

Table 14.1 Factors influencing the results of the exercise ECG stress test.

Methods
Exercise protocol
ECG lead system
Criteria to terminate exercise
Interpretation
Diagnostic criteria utilized
Diagnosis of arrhythmias
Population
Prevalence of CAD in population
Factors for False-Positive/False-Negative Tests

The literature frequently uses the terms "sensitivity," "specificity," and "predictive value" when assessing diagnostic studies. Exercise ECG stress testing is reported to have a mean sensitivity and specificity of 68% and 77%, respectively, for the diagnosis of CAD. As highlighted in Chapter 3, the sensitivity and specificity of the exercise ECG test will vary with the diagnostic criteria used for a positive test as well as the definition of "hemodynamically significant" CAD used during coronary angiography. Bayes' theorem dictates that positive and negative predictive valves will vary with the incidence of CAD in the population being tested. For example, the positive predictive value will decline if a population of asymptomatic healthy individuals are referred for testing as the incidence of CAD in this population is quite low.

This chapter will review the normal and abnormal physiologic responses to exercise as well as the interpretation of electrocardiographic changes during exercise.

Physiologic Responses to Exercise

Various physiologic responses to exercise are expected in healthy individuals (Table 14.2).

BP and HR Changes

- Progressive increases in HR and systolic blood pressure (SBP) with exercise are expected in healthy individuals.
- For patients in sinus rhythm, a linear increase in HR is expected with increasing workload and oxygen demand.

Table 14.2 Expected physiologic responses to exercise.

Progressive increase in HR and BP
Shortening of the QT interval
Physiologic ST-segment alterations
Functional (J-point) ST-segment depression with duration less than 60–80 ms
Orthostatic ECG changes
Labile T-wave change
Reynold's syndrome
Alteration of T-wave direction or morphology
Decrease in R-wave amplitude
Shortening of PR-interval
Downward sloping of PR-segment
Decrease in T-wave amplitude in early exercise, followed by increase in T-wave amplitude

- HR is generally expected to increase by 10 bpm per metabolic equivalent (MET). A rapid rise in HR can be seen in patients with decreased physical conditioning, metabolic disorders, variable vascular volume or peripheral resistance, anemia, or ventricular dysfunction. A slow rise in HR may be seen in healthy patients with excellent physical conditioning or among patients with sinus node dysfunction, chronotropic incompetence, or in patients taking atrioventricular (AV) nodal blocking agents such as beta-blockers or non-dihydropyridine calcium channel blockers.
- The maximal HR achieved with exercise is influenced by a number of factors. Expected maximal HR can be predicted by use of several different equations; in our laboratory we utilize the formula:
  - Age-predicted maximal HR = 220 bpm − age (yrs).
  - 85% of this value is one commonly used criterion to define satisfactory effort during exercise testing.
  - It must be appreciated that a variability exists (±12 bpm) when considering what the maximal HR may be for any particular individual.
- A rapid decline in HR is expected during the first 30 seconds of recovery, followed by a gradual return to baseline, reflecting normal vagal activity. Often referred to as heart rate recovery (HRR), this finding has gained increased attention and studies have suggested that an abnormal HRR response is a predictor of increased mortality.
- Systolic BP increases progressively with exercise as a result of increased cardiac output (Q), generally about 10 mmHg/MET. In contrast with the SBP response to exercise, DBP is generally unchanged or slightly decreased due to increased vasodilation. An increase in SBP beyond 210 mmHg in men and 190 mmHg in women is considered an abnormal response.
- After cessation of exercise, SBP declines due to a decrease in Q. When exercise is abruptly terminated without a cool down period, some healthy patients may experience a rapid drop in BP due to a combination of rapid reduction in Q, increased venous pooling, and persistent vasodilation.

Alteration of the QT-Interval

- In general, the QT-interval is expected to shorten during exercise due to a shortened action potential with increases in HR. Paradoxically, some patients, more commonly women, may experience a prolongation of the QT-interval during early exercise.
- The Bazett corrected QT-interval (QTc) commonly increases at low workloads and subsequently decreases at higher workloads.
- Purported measurements that have assessed QT-interval responses to exercise as predictive of underlying CAD are found to have limited value.

Physiologic ST-Segment Alteration

- The J-junction, also known as J-point, represents the end of the QRS complex and the beginning of the ST-segment.
- The J-point can be depressed at maximum exercise in healthy patients. Therefore, the magnitude of ST-segment depression should be measured 60–80 ms after the J-point.
- Upsloping ST-segment depression at peak exercise may be seen in 10–20% of normal patients.
- Non-specific ST-segment and T-wave abnormalities in the resting ECG limits the ability to interpret the exercise ECG.

Variations of T-Wave Morphology

- Alterations in T-wave morphology are common during exercise.
- T-wave amplitude tends to decrease in early exercise, but tends to return to baseline values at higher workloads. In the early recovery period, T-wave amplitude may increase further.

- Although at one time tall T-waves during exercise were considered indicative for subendocardial ischemia, this is no longer accepted. Many healthy and young individuals demonstrate tall T-waves during exercise and in recovery.
- Previously, myocardial ischemia was diagnosed when inverted T-waves became upright during or after exercise. At present, this finding is of unclear clinical significance.

Changes in QRS Morphology and Amplitude

- In healthy subjects, the QRS duration decreases at higher workloads as a result of increased conduction velocity within the heart.
- The total amplitude of the QRS is reduced slightly during near maximal exercise
- An increase in magnitude of septal Q waves in lateral leads is also expected, as is a decrease in R-wave and S-wave amplitudes in the inferior leads.
- The Athens QRS score incorporates changes in Q, R, and S-wave amplitudes into a score that can be used for diagnostic purposes.

Alterations of the P-wave and PR-Interval

- P-wave amplitude increases during exercise, while the duration of the P-wave is minimally affected.
- Physiologic shortening of the PR-interval is observed soon after the initiation of exercise.
- Downward displacement of the PR-segment can occur during exercise as the P-wave becomes taller and the T-a wave (atrial repolarization wave) becomes prominent. When this occurs, the T-a wave tends to extend through the QRS complex, and may alter the junction between the ST-segment and the T-wave, resulting in apparent ST-segment depression.

Abnormal Responses to Exercise

There are three major abnormal responses that may be elicited during an exercise ECG test (Table 14.3).

- Electrical events: ECG changes: ST-segment depression or elevation and various arrhythmias.
- Hemodynamic events: alterations in BP and HR.
- Symptomatic manifestations and signs.

Among these ischemic responses, alterations of the ST-segment are the most widely accepted criteria for the diagnosis of myocardial ischemia. The diagnostic accuracy is increased when ST-segment alterations are interpreted in conjunction with other signs of ischemia, such as chest pain or abnormal BP response. Accuracy is also increased when exercise ECG testing is performed in conjunction with myocardial imaging (see Chapters 6 and 7), particularly in the presence of left bundle branch block (LBBB), left ventricular hypertrophy (LVH) with repolarization abnormality, ventricular pacing, Wolff-Parkinson-White (WPW) pattern, digitalis effect, and other conditions known to affect repolarization.

There are numerous factors that may influence the result of the exercise ECG test. Chapter 15 will review the many factors can produce false-positive (Table 14.4) or false-negative results (Table 14.5). There is a higher incidence of false-positive exercise ECG tests in women. While some have advocated for the addition of myocardial imaging in female patients, the WOMEN trial found similar two-year outcomes among patients undergoing exercise ECG vs. exercise myocardial perfusion imaging (MPI).

The sensitivity of the exercise ECG test varies with the number of coronary vessels involved. The sensitivity for detecting single-vessel CAD is low (37–60%), with a significant increase (86–100%) when three vessels are involved. In two-vessel disease, sensitivity ranges from 67–91%.

Table 14.3 Abnormal responses to exercise.

Electrocardiographic changes

    Diagnostic ST-segment alterations

        ST-segment depression (horizontal or downsloping)

        ST-segment elevation (without prior MI)

        Additional ST-segment change with pre-existing ECG abnormalities

    Significant arrhythmias

    Inversion of U-waves

    Intraventricular blocks (not diagnostic for CAD)

    Increased R-wave amplitude

    Acute MI

Hemodynamic changes

    Hypotension/blunted BP response

    Slowing of HR

    Impaired HR response

    Marked hypertension

Signs and symptoms

    Signs: Third or fourth heart sounds, murmurs, precordial bulging, double cardiac impulse, pulses alternans

    Symptoms: angina, dyspnea, pallor, cyanosis, syncope, etc.

Table 14.4 Factors that may result in false-positive exercise ECG tests.

Medications

Digitalis, diuretics, anti-depressants, sedatives, estrogen

Cardiac disorders

Wolff-Parkinson-White (WPW) syndrome

Cardiomyopathies including hypertrophic cardiomyopathy

LVH including hypertensive heart disease

Myocarditis and pericarditis

Rheumatic heart disease

Electrolyte imbalances

Hypokalemia

Pre-existing ECG abnormalities

LVH with repolarization abnormality

Left bundle branch block

Ventricular pacing

Nonspecific ST-T abnormalities ($\geq$0.5–1.0 mm ST-segment depression)

Wolf-Parkinson-White pattern/syndrome

Table 14.5 Factors that may result in false-negative exercise ECG tests.

Medications

  Beta-blockers, calcium channel blockers, nitrates, and other anti-anginal medications, procainamide, quinidine, phenothiazines

Inadequate exercise

  Submaximal exercise

  Premature termination of testing

  Improper lead system

Miscellaneous

  Coronary artery disease of borderline severity

  Left axis deviation, left anterior fascicular block

Electrocardiographic Changes

Among various ECG changes induced by exercise, the most reliable diagnostic finding suggestive of obstructive CAD is the horizontal or downsloping ST segment depression of 1 mm or more at 60–80 ms after the J-point (measured relative to the PQ-segment). Specific exercise-induced arrhythmias, such as multifocal ventricular premature contraction (VPCs), grouped (three or more) VPCs, and ventricular tachycardia (VT), may be predictive of CAD when associated with ST-segment changes or chest pain. Frequent or complex ventricular ectopy, particularly in the recovery period, has been associated with increased risk for death. Other findings, such as inverted U-waves (a very uncommon occurrence) or increased R-wave amplitude may also be suggestive of myocardial ischemia. Table 14.6 summarizes criteria for a positive exercise ECG stress test.

Table 14.6 Criteria for positive exercise ECG stress test.

Horizontal or downsloping ST-segment depression of ≥1 mm at 60–80 ms during or after exercise
Upsloping ST segment depression ≥2 mm 80 ms beyond the J-point during or after exercise (may be considered an equivocal response)
ST segment elevation ≥1 mm during or after exercise in the absence of Q waves
Exercise-induced hypotension
Inversion of U-waves
Frequent multifocal ventricular premature contraction (VPCs), grouped (three or more) VPCs, ventricular tachycardia (VT) at low-exercise workload
Exercise-induced typical angina
Third or fourth heart sounds, or heart murmur

Diagnostic ST-Segment Alterations

ST-Segment Depression

- ST depression during exercise represents ischemia induced electrical gradients across the endocardium and epicardium. ST depression can be upsloping, horizontal, or downsloping (Figure 14.1).
- It is important to note ST-segment depression during exercise does not reliably localize ischemia to a specific coronary vessel.
- Factors that relate to the probability and severity of CAD include the severity, onset, duration/regression, and number of leads with ST-segment depression.

ST SEGMENT DEPRESSION DURING EXERCISE

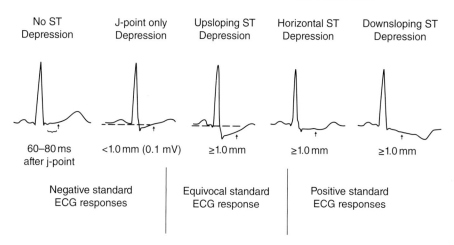

Figure 14.1 Types of ST depression seen during exercise. *Source:* Reproduced, with permission, from Fletcher et al. (2013).

- Traditionally, ≥1 mm of horizontal or downsloping ST segment depression in three consecutive beats during or after exercise has been considered the most reliable diagnostic criteria of myocardial ischemia (Figure 14.2).
- Upsloping ST-segment depression of ≥2 mm at 60–80 ms beyond the J-point has been considered by some investigators to be suggestive of myocardial ischemia; however, this finding should more correctly be considered to be an "equivocal" response. Both "rapid" and "slow" upsloping of the ST-segment with exercise have been shown to be

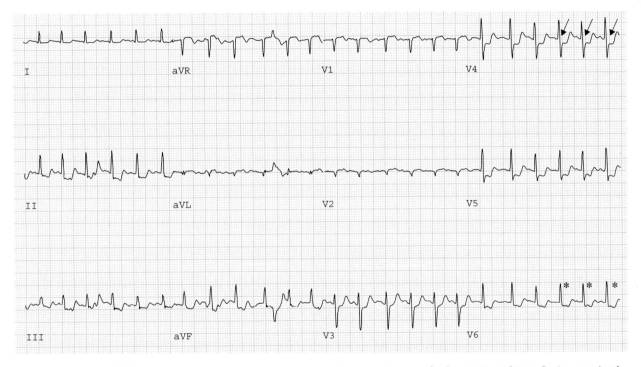

Figure 14.2 Exercise ECG in a 64-year-old male referred for exercise testing for evaluation of a chest pain syndrome. During exercise the patient developed up to 2 mm of horizontal (arrow) and downsloping (asterisk) ST-segment depression that persisted well into the recovery phase. Coronary angiography demonstrated severe three-vessel coronary artery disease.

associated with a low incidence of myocardial ischemia with SPECT-MPI and transient ischemic dilatation of the LV. Interestingly, initial upsloping ST-segment depression can be followed by horizontal or downsloping ST-segment depression (Figures 14.3 and 14.4) at slower HRs; this response should be considered as one indicative of CAD.

- Minor upsloping ST-depression, whether rapid or slow, has not been reliably predictive of the presence of myocardial ischemia as it is comparably prevalent in patients with and without CAD. Therefore, this response is generally defined as equivocal (Figure 14.5).
- Diagnostic ST-segment depression associated with frequent VPCs, multifocal VPCs, or grouped beats is suggestive of advanced CAD with multivessel involvement (Figure 14.6).

Several caveats concerning ST-segment depression during and/or after exercise should be particularly emphasized:

- Time of onset and regression of ST-segment change:
  - Horizontal or downsloping ST-segment depression beginning at low exercise workloads and persisting for several minutes into the recovery period, is highly suggestive of underlying advanced CAD.
  - Persistence of ST-segment depression beyond two to three minutes in the recovery period is more indicative of an ischemic response to exercise than a false-positive result.
  - Rapid resolution of ST-segment depression in the recovery period (within 60 seconds), especially when other high-risk indicators are absent, is associated with low-risk for future atherosclerotic cardiovascular disease (ASCVD) events and no significant benefit from further diagnostic testing.
- Recovery-only ST-segment depression:
  - ST-segment depression found only in the recovery period, which occurs in approximately 8–10% of patients with abnormal ST-segment responses to exercise, carries the same diagnostic implications as ST-segment depression that develops during exercise.

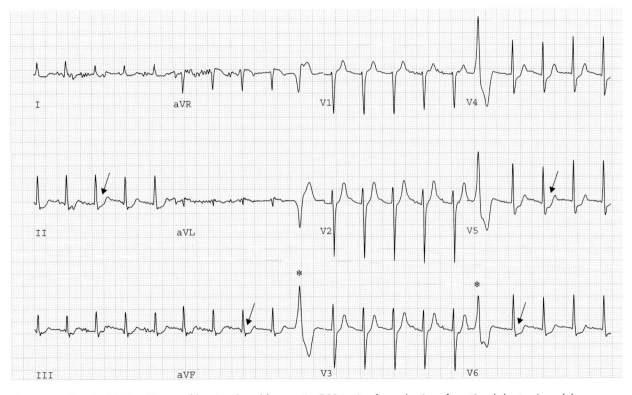

Figure 14.3 Exercise ECG in a 58-year-old male referred for exercise ECG testing for evaluation of exertional chest pain and dyspnea. Note the slow-upsloping ST depression (arrows), measuring up to 2 mm, and ventricular premature contractions (asterisks).

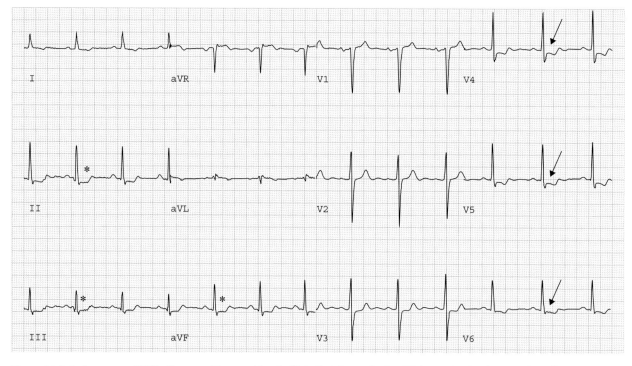

Figure 14.4 Early recovery ECG in the same 58-year-old male. Note that the upsloping ST depression has been replaced by horizontal (asterisks) and downsloping (arrows) ST-depression during the recovery phase.

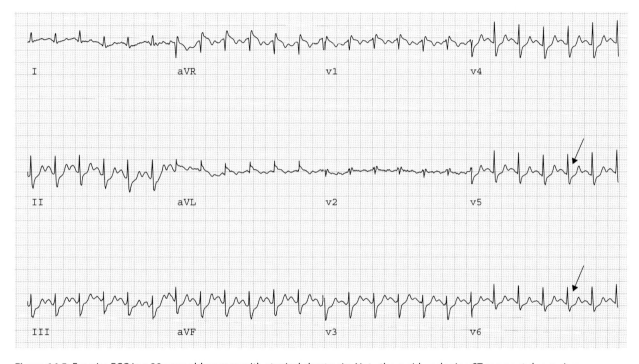

Figure 14.5 Exercise ECG in a 38-year-old woman with atypical chest pain. Note the rapid-upsloping ST-segment depression. Echocardiographic images immediately following the exercise bout did not demonstrate new wall motion abnormalities to suggest ischemia.

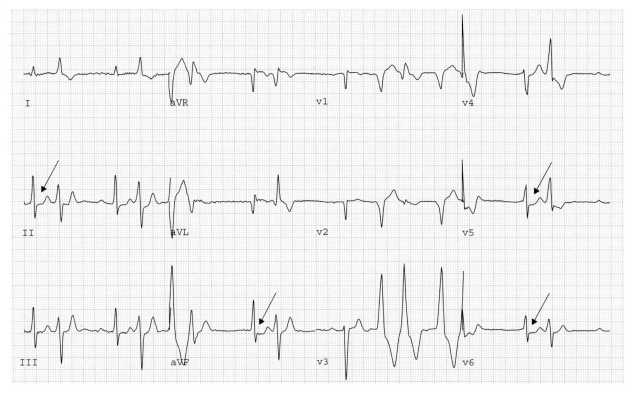

Figure 14.6 Recovery ECG in a 75-year-old male with known coronary artery disease (CAD) undergoing exercise testing for new exertional chest pain. Frequent ventricular premature contractions (VPCs) in couplets and triplets are present. Note associated ST-segment depression in inferolateral leads indicative of ischemia (arrows). At coronary angiography, the patient was found to have severe three-vessel CAD.

- Particular leads involved:
  - ST-segment depression localized only to the inferior leads has been shown to be an unreliable marker for the diagnosis of CAD compared to ST-segment depression occurring in lead V5 or in both V5 *and* inferior leads.

ST-Segment Elevation

- ST-segment elevation in the absence of pre-existing Q-waves during exercise is rarely encountered in patients with normal resting ECGs. It can be encountered in patients with coronary artery spasm or those with significant sub-total occlusive CAD.
- J point/ST-segment elevation at rest is commonly encountered in healthy young individuals and returns to isoelectric during exercise and reappears during the recovery period.
- ST-segment elevation of ≥1 mm in the absence of prior Q waves (excepting leads aVR, V1, and aVL) is strongly suggestive of transmural myocardial ischemia. This finding localizes ischemia to a specific coronary vessel, often with an underlying, high-grade lesion being found at coronary angiography (Figure 14.7).
- ST-segment elevation can occur during exercise testing in leads with pre-existing Q waves and may represent peri-infarct ischemia, ventricular dyskinesis, or akinetic myocardium. This finding can be seen in up to 30% of patients with prior anterior MI and 15% of patients with prior inferior MI. Imaging may demonstrate ventricular aneurysm (Figure 14.8).
- Development of 1 mm of ST-segment elevation, 60 ms after the J point is considered an abnormal response in patients with pre-existing Q waves. Reciprocal ST depression may accompany ST-segment elevation.

ST-Segment Alterations with Preexisting ECG Abnormalities

- The exercise ECG is challenging to interpret when nonspecific ST-segment and T-wave abnormalities are present at baseline.

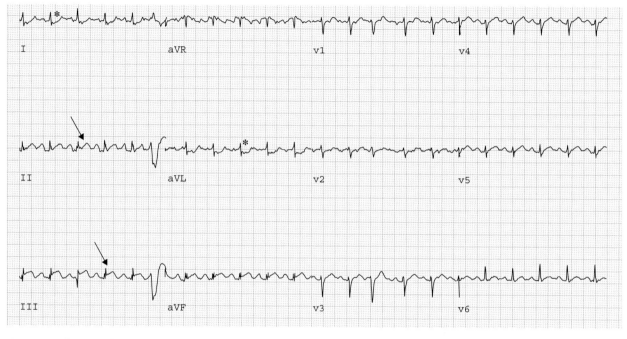

Figure 14.7 Exercise ECG in a 70-year-old woman with chest pain and dyspnea. Note the inferior ST-segment elevation (arrows) and lateral ST-segment depression (asterisk). Coronary angiography demonstrated an occluded mid-right coronary artery which with prominent septal collaterals from the left anterior descending artery.

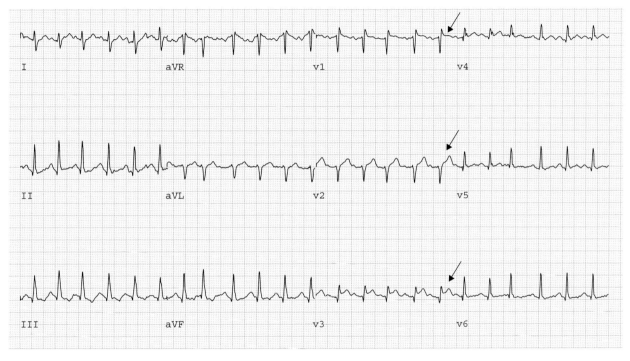

Figure 14.8 Exercise ECG in a 70-year-old male with known anteroseptal infarction. Note the ST-segment elevation in anterior leads which also contain Q-waves (arrows). Echocardiography demonstrated an akinetic anterior wall, while coronary angiography showed a widely patent left internal mammary artery (LIMA) graft supplying the left anterior descending artery.

- In the setting of baseline ST-T abnormalities, an additional 1 mm of ST-segment depression is considered an abnormal response, although the specificity of these findings is reduced (Figures 14.9–14.12).
- Resting ST-T abnormalities are often due to LVH with repolarization abnormality (Figures 14.13 and 14.14), LBBB, or ventricular pacing. When LVH with repolarization abnormality, LBBB, or ventricular pacing are present, the exercise ECG is not interpretable for myocardial ischemia, and testing must be performed in conjunction with myocardial imaging (see Chapter 11).
- When a right bundle branch block (RBBB) is present, the exercise ECG can be interpreted, although exaggerated ST segment depression in leads V2–3 may be anticipated (Figures 14.15–14.16).

Cardiac Arrhythmias

Various arrhythmias may be provoked or suppressed with exercise in healthy individuals. These are reviewed in detail in Chapter 12.

- Frequent VPCs, multifocal VPCs, grouped VPCs, and VT provoked at low workloads are suggestive of underlying CAD, particularly if ST-segment depression is present in other beats (Figure 14.6).
- Marked bradycardia may occur in patients with advanced CAD during the immediate post-exercise period, and can be associated with angina, hypotension, and significant ST-segment depression.

Inversion of U Waves

Although rare, exercise-induced U-wave inversion in patients with a normal resting ECG can be suggestive of single-vessel CAD of the left anterior descending artery (LAD).

Intraventricular Blocks

Exercise-induced intraventricular blocks are discussed in detail in Chapter 12. Various intraventricular blocks including LBBB, RBBB, fascicular blocks, and bifascicular blocks may be observed during or after exercise; they usually represent a rate-dependent phenomenon and therefore, are not diagnostic for myocardial ischemia.

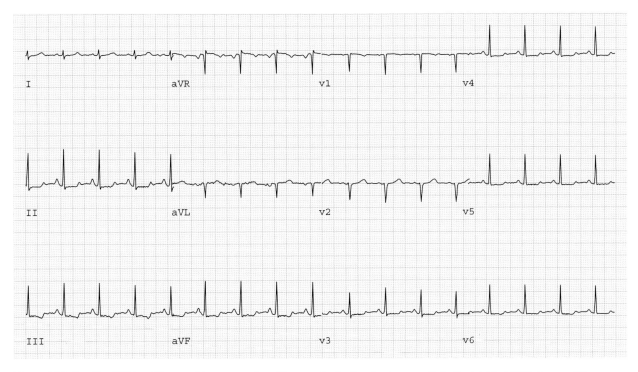

Figure 14.9 Baseline ECG in a 38-year-old woman referred for exercise testing for dyspnea. Note the baseline ST-T abnormalities.

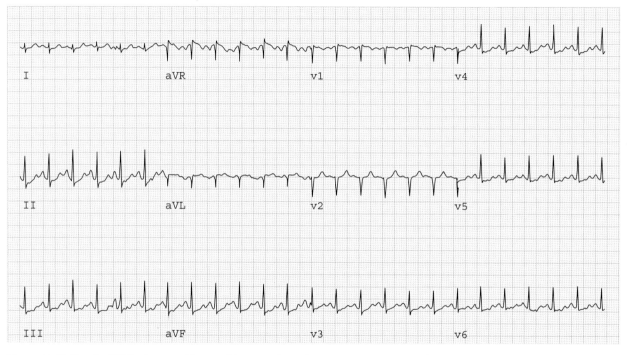

Figure 14.10 Exercise ECG in the same 38-year-old woman. Note the persistent ST segment depression during exercise. Concurrent echocardiography did not demonstrate evidence of inducible ischemia.

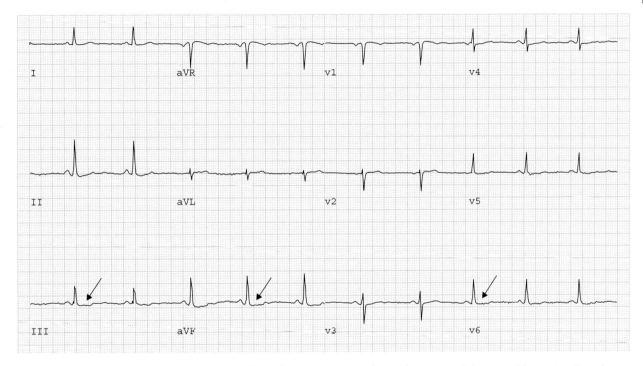

Figure 14.11 Baseline ECG in a 57-year-old male referred for exercise testing due to chest pain and dyspnea with exertion. Note the mild baseline ST-segment depression (arrows).

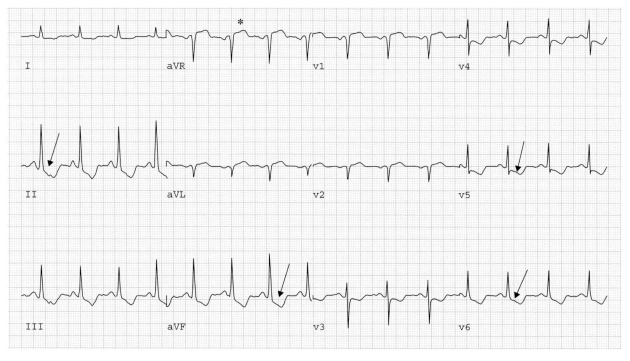

Figure 14.12 Recovery ECG in the same 57-year-old male. Note the marked diffuse downsloping ST-segment depression (arrows) and ST-segment elevation in lead aVR (asterisk). ECG changes began by 1 minute of exercise and resolved after 12 minutes of recovery. Concurrent echocardiographic imaging demonstrated inducible ischemia in multiple vascular territories. Coronary angiography demonstrated severe three-vessel coronary artery disease.

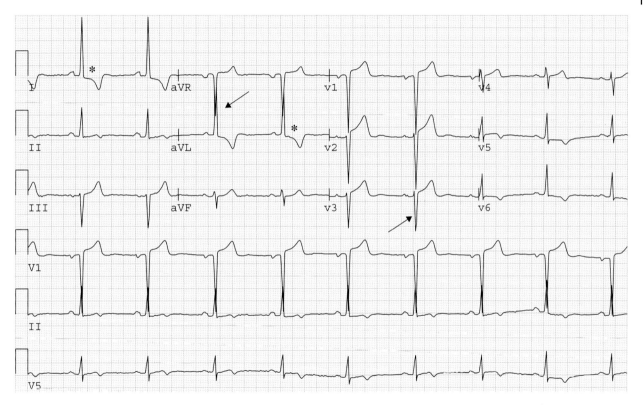

Figure 14.13 Baseline ECG in a 66-year-old woman with aortic stenosis demonstrating LVH (arrows) with repolarization abnormalitles (asterisk).

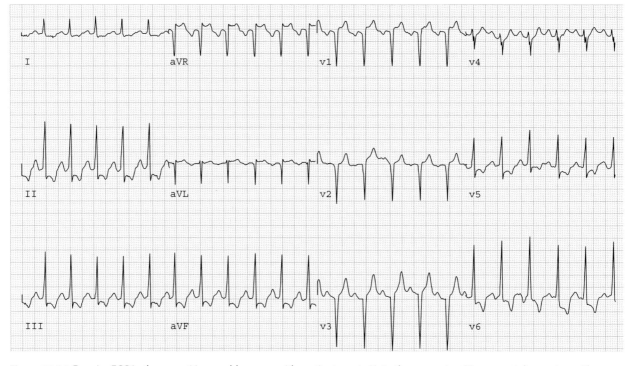

Figure 14.14 Exercise ECG in the same 66-year-old woman with aortic stenosis. Note the worsening ST-segment depression with exercise. Pre-operative coronary angiography did not demonstrate obstructive coronary artery disease.

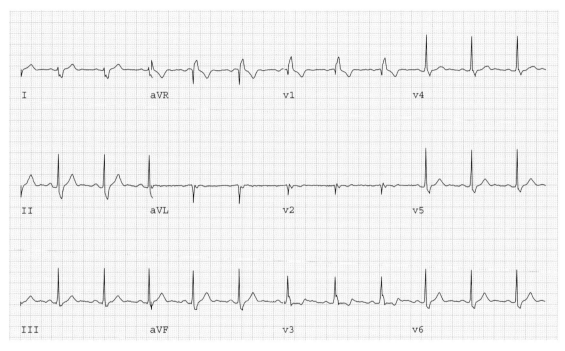

Figure 14.15 Baseline ECG demonstrating right bundle branch block (RBBB) in a 56-year-old male referred for exercise testing for atypical chest pain.

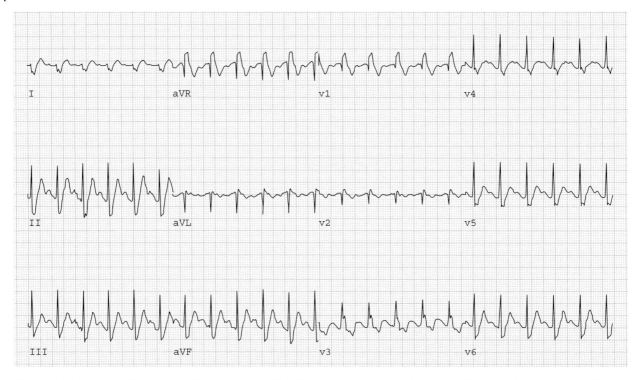

Figure 14.16 Exercise ECG in the same 56-year-old male. Note the persistent ST depression in leads V1–3 associated with the RBBB, but normal ST-segments in other leads. This exercise ECG was interpreted as normal and no perfusion defects were noted on myocardial perfusion imaging (MPI).

Increased R-Wave Amplitude

The amplitude of the QRS complex generally increases during submaximal exercise and decreases during maximum exercise. Some investigators emphasize that an increase in QRS amplitude at peak exercise has been associated with myocardial ischemia, possibly reflecting LV ischemic dilation.

P-Wave Abnormalities

Increases in P-wave duration and P-wave amplitude during exercise have been reported to be greater in patients with reversible perfusion defects on MPI when compared with patients with normal perfusion. This may be related to an increase in left atrial pressure during ischemia.

Hemodynamic Changes

Myocardial oxygen demand and consumption increases with exercise. To meet these needs, Q is augmented through an increase in SV and HR. As previously described, an incremental increase in HR and SBP is expected during exercise. When augmentation in HR and/or blood BP fails to occur with progressive exercise, abnormal hemodynamic alterations should be considered.

Hypotension

- A decline in SBP below resting value at the onset of exercise-induced angina is suggestive of multivessel CAD.
- A reduction in SBP below resting values in the absence of angina can also be encountered in patients with severe valvular heart disease, LV outflow tract obstruction due to hypertrophic cardiomyopathy or multivessel CAD.
- Pharmacological stress agents may reduce Q or systemic vascular resistance, resulting in transient hypotension.

Abnormal HR Response

- A progressive acceleration of HR is expected during multistage ECG testing, although physically active individuals, such as trained athletes, may not exhibit the expected HR acceleration during exercise.
- Failure of the increment in HR during exercise (chronotropic incompetence) may be an important abnormal response to exercise and may be reflective of underlying CAD or sick sinus syndrome when occurring in the absence of AV nodal blocking agents, such as beta-blockers or non-dihydropyridine calcium channel blockers.

Marked Hypertension

An increase in SBP beyond 210 mmHg in men and 190 mmHg in women during exercise is considered an abnormal response and can be suggestive of labile hypertension. Exercise ECG testing should be terminated when SBP exceeds 250 mmHg and/or DBP is greater than 115 mmHg.

Symptoms and Signs

A variety of symptoms and signs may be observed during exercise testing.

Symptoms

- Symptoms such as fatigue and dyspnea are common.
- Chest pain can occur during exercise testing and it is important to understand if the chest pain is similar that which prompted testing.
- Typical angina, reproducible with exercise, is predictive of CAD, especially if accompanied by ST-segment depression.

- Atypical chest pain or nonspecific chest pain lacks reproducibility. In many cases, atypical chest pain cannot be reproduced at workloads that exceed those experienced during index symptoms.
- Severe dyspnea, marked pallor, cyanosis, syncope, or near syncope are abnormal responses to exercise.

Signs

- A clearly audible S4 provoked by exercise can be suggestive of inducible LV dysfunction.
- An audible S3 provoked by exercise may be suggestive of advanced CAD and/or LV dysfunction.
- Systolic murmurs induced by exercise may represent mitral regurgitation due to ischemia-induced papillary muscle dysfunction.
- Other abnormal signs may include exercise-induced pulsus alternans, abnormal precordial bulges, and palpable thrills.

Clinical Implications

The exercise ECG is an important noninvasive method for evaluating chest pain syndromes and diagnosing CAD. As previously noted, it has excellent sensitivity for the diagnosis of three-vessel disease, but modest sensitivity for the diagnosis of single-vessel disease.

In addition to evaluating chest pain syndromes, exercise-induced arrhythmias, and diagnosing CAD, exercise ECG testing is helpful in evaluating exercise capacity as well as the efficacy of medical therapy. Exercise ECG testing also allows patients to be grouped into functional classes based on METs achieved (see Table 3.3).

Importantly, the exercise ECG also provides significant prognostic information.

- The Duke Treadmill Score (DTS), the most commonly used index, predicts mortality risk based on diagnostic parameters met during exercise, including duration of exercise, severity of ST-segment depression, and treadmill anginal index:

$$DTS = \text{Exercise Time (in min)} - 5 \times \textit{maximal ST-segment deviation} \text{ (in mm)} - 4 \times \text{anginal index}$$

  where no angina = 0, non-limiting angina = 1, and limiting angina = 2.

- Patients are grouped into low (DTS ≥ +5), moderate (DTS –10 to +4) and high-risk (≤ –11) categories. Overall five-year survival has been found to be 95% in the low-risk group, 90% in the moderate-risk group, and 65% in the high-risk group.

Reporting

The exercise ECG report should include:

- The method of testing (exercise vs pharmacological) as well as the protocol utilized.
- Signs and symptoms (e.g. chest pain) that developed during and/or after exercise as well as the reason for test termination.
- The findings of the baseline (standard) 12-lead ECG.
- Stage at which exercise was terminated, maximal HR, including percentage of maximal age-predicted HR, and maximal BP.
- HR and BP response (normal or abnormal).
- ST-segment changes in response to exercise. These should be discussed in detail – stage, HR, persistence in recovery, number of leads involved, and double product of onset and resolution.

- Arrhythmias that were provoked during or after exercise.
- Functional classification and METs achieved.
- Duke treadmill score.
- Post-exercise HRR.
- Description as to whether the test is positive, negative, non-diagnostic, or borderline/equivocal.
- Indicate if testing should be repeated.
- If testing is canceled, reasoning should be described.
- If scheduled testing is not desirable, alternative testing modalities should be advised along with the reasoning.

Summary

- The exercise ECG stress test is an important non-invasive tool in the diagnosis of CAD and evaluating chest pain syndromes.
- Results should be interpreted in the context of a patient's history, physical examination, resting 12-lead ECG, and other laboratory and imaging data.
- Three major myocardial ischemic responses to exercise may occur: electrocardiographic changes, abnormal hemodynamic response(s), and symptom development.
- Physiologic and abnormal responses to exercise are summarized in Tables 14.2 and 14.3.
- Horizontal or downsloping ST-segment depression ≥1 mm at 60–80 ms after the J-point is generally accepted as an abnormal finding suggestive of myocardial ischemia. Upsloping ST-segment depression (rapid or slow morphology) represents an equivocal response.
- ST-segment depression evoked with exercise does not serve to localize ischemia to a specific coronary vessel territory.

- ST-segment elevation may occur during exercise testing in leads with pre-existing Q waves. This finding can be seen in up to 30% of patients with prior anterior MI and 15% of patients with prior inferior MI and may represent peri-infarct ischemia, ventricular dyskinesis, or akinetic myocardium.
- ST-segment elevation is an uncommon finding with stress testing in leads without pre-existing Q-waves. In this situation, its occurrence often indicates the presence of transmural myocardial ischemia due to a significant, usually proximal, underlying coronary artery lesion. This finding localizes ischemia to the specific vascular territory involved.
- The presence of ventricular arrhythmias, including frequent VPCs, multifocal VPCs, grouped VPCs, and VT at low workloads, is highly suspicious for CAD, especially when accompanied by an abnormal ST-segment response or chest pain.
- Development of exercise-induced hypotension and typical angina is highly suspicious for the diagnosis of CAD.
- Functional classification of patients can be determined on the basis of the achieved exercise workload, expressed in METs.
- The exercise ECG test also carries important prognostic implications. The DTS, the most commonly used exercise ECG index, permits categorization of patients into low, moderate, and high-risk groups based on three exercise ECG test variables.

References

Christman, M.P., Bittencourt, M.S., Hulten, E. et al. (2014). Yield of downstream tests after exercise treadmill testing: a prospective cohort study. *J. Am. Coll. Cardiol.* 63: 1264–1274.

Cole, C.R., Blackstone, E.H., Pashkow, F.J. et al. (1999). Heart-rate recovery immediately after exercise as a predictor of mortality. *N. Engl. J. Med.* 341: 1351–1357.

Desai, M.Y., Crugnale, S., Mondeau, J. et al. (2002). Slow upsloping ST-segment depression during exercise: does it really signify a positive stress test? *Am. Heart J.* 143: 482–487.

Fletcher, G.F., Ades, P.A., Kligfield, P. et al., on behalf of the American Heart Association Exercise, Cardiac Rehabilitation, and Prevention Committee of the Council on Clinical Cardiology, Council on Nutrition, Physical Activity and Metabolism, Council on Cardiovascular and Stroke Nursing, and Council on Epidemiology and Prevention (2013). Exercise standards for testing and training: a scientific statement from the American Heart Association. *Circulation* 128: 873–934.

Garber, A.M. and Solomon, N.A. (1999). Cost-effectiveness of alternative test strategies for the diagnosis of coronary artery disease. *Ann. Intern. Med.* 130: 719–728.

Gibbons, R.J. (2002). Abnormal heart-rate recovery after exercise. *Lancet* 259: 1536–1537.

Goldschlager, N., Selzer, A., and Cohn, K. (1976). Treadmill stress tests as indicators of presence and severity of coronary artery disease. *Ann. Intern. Med.* 85: 277–286.

Kligfield, P., Ameisen, O., and Okin, P.M. (1989). Heart rate adjustment of ST segment depression for improved detection of coronary artery disease. *Circulation* 79: 245–255.

Kodama, K., Hiasa, G., Ohtsuka, T. et al. (2000). Transient U wave inversion during treadmill exercise testing in patients with left anterior descending coronary artery disease. *Angiology* 51: 581–589.

Lachterman, B., Lehmann, K.G., Abrahamson, D., and Froelicher, V.F. (1990). "Recovery only" ST-segment depression and the predictive accuracy of the exercise test. *Ann. Intern. Med.* 112: 11–16. Erratum in: Ann. Intern. Med. 1990; 113: 333–334.

Mark, D.B., Hlatky, M.A., Harrell, F.E. Jr. et al. (1987). Exercise treadmill score for predicting prognosis in coronary artery disease. *Ann. Intern. Med.* 106: 793–800.

Michaelides, A.P., Triposkiadis, F.K., Boudoulas, H. et al. (1990). New coronary artery disease index based on exercise-induced QRS changes. *Am. Heart J.* 120: 292–302.

Miranda, C.P., Liu, J., Kadar, A. et al. (1992). Usefulness of exercise-induced ST-segment depression in the inferior leads during exercise testing as a marker for coronary artery disease. *Am. J. Cardiol.* 69: 303–307.

Shaw, L.J., Peterson, E.D., Shaw, L.K. et al. (1998). Use of a prognostic treadmill score in identifying diagnostic coronary disease subgroups. *Circulation* 98: 1622–1630.

Shaw, L.J., Mieres, J.H., Hendel, R.H. et al., WOMEN Trial Investigators (2011). Comparative effectiveness of exercise electrocardiography with or without myocardial perfusion single photon emission computed tomography in women with suspected coronary artery disease: results from the What Is the Optimal Method for Ischemia Evaluation in Women (WOMEN) trial. *Circulation* 124: 1239–1249.

15 False-Positive and False-Negative Exercise ECG Test Results

John B. Dickey

Introduction

As with all medical testing, the exercise stress ECG test is not without inaccuracy for the detection of coronary artery disease (CAD). False-positive (exercise-induced ST-segment depression in the absence of significant epicardial CAD) and false-negative (lack of exercise-induced ST-segment depression in the presence of significant epicardial CAD) results occur and cannot be avoided completely. In meta-analyses, using horizontal or down-sloping ST segment deviation of ≥1 mm persistent 80 ms after the J-point as the criterion for abnormal response, the exercise stress ECG test has been shown to have a mean sensitivity of 68% and mean specificity of 77% for the detection of CAD. Numerous factors can lead to false-positive and false-negative results, including use of medications, conduction system disease, Left ventricular hypertrophy (LVH) and other conditions that affect repolarization, valvular heart disease, gender, and testing equipment. In this chapter, the various factors leading to false-positive or false-negative ECG responses to exercise will be discussed (Table 15.1).

Pocket Guide to Stress Testing, Second Edition. Edited by Dennis A. Tighe and Bryon A. Gentile.
© 2020 John Wiley & Sons Ltd. Published 2020 by John Wiley & Sons Ltd.

Table 15.1 Causes of False-Positive and False-Negative Exercise ECG Results.

False-Positive	False-Negative
• Digitalis use	• Submaximal stress workload
• Mitral valve prolapse/regurgitation	• Beta-adrenergic blockers
• Left ventricular hypertrophy	• Calcium channel blockers
• Left bundle branch block	• Nitrates
• Ventricular pacing	• L-arginine
• Ventricular pre-excitation (Wolff-Parkinson-White [WPW] syndrome or pattern)	• Single vessel coronary artery disease (circumflex territory)
• Hypokalemia with ST-segment changes	• Coronary artery disease of borderline significance
• ≥0.5–1.0 mm resting ST-segment depression	
• Female gender	
• Computer-aided post processing	
• Atrial repolarization (Ta) wave	

False-Positive Exercise ECG Responses

Digitalis

- The cardiac glycoside digitalis is a well-known cause of abnormalities in the resting ECG. The "digitalis effect" is described as a sagging or down-sloping depression of the ST-segment accompanied by shortening of the QT-interval. However, resting ECG abnormalities may not be present in every patient taking digitalis.

- During exercise, digitalis will accentuate ST-segment deviation due to ischemia in patients with CAD and can cause ST-segment depression both during and after exercise in 25–40% of normal healthy subjects. Resting ECG abnormalities due to digitalis effect will be accentuated with exercise.
- Although ST-segment deviation due to digitalis uncommonly exceeds 2 mm, it is difficult to differentiate the false-positive response to digitalis from the true positive response to ischemia; marked ST-segment deviation (>3–4 mm) should prompt consideration that the response may be a true positive.
- A negative exercise ECG stress test in a digitalized patient suggests against the presence of CAD.
- Cardiac arrhythmias due to digitalis can be exacerbated with exercise and therefore suspected digitalis toxicity is a relative contraindication to stress testing.
- While digitalis remains in the circulation for several weeks after discontinuation, ECG effects typically resolve in 90% of patients within 7–10 days after withdrawal.

Mitral Valve Prolapse/Mitral Regurgitation

- Patients with MVP have a higher incidence of ST-segment changes on exercise ECG testing, which may be exacerbated with greater degrees of mitral regurgitation.
- The exact mechanism for this phenomenon is not fully understood, but proposed mechanisms include abnormalities of the coronary arteries, coronary vasospasm, concomitant cardiomyopathy, regional ischemia of the papillary muscles, or coronary artery compression.
- Given this potential effect on the ECG response to exercise, patients with known MVP or more than moderate mitral regurgitation should be considered for exercise ECG testing with concomitant myocardial imaging.

Left Ventricular Hypertrophy

- Patients with voltage criteria for LVH accompanied by ST-T abnormalities, consistent with a "strain pattern," have a high incidence of false-positive exercise ECG changes, even when the ST-segment deviation is marked (>2 mm).

- Similar false-positive changes can be seen in patients with voltage criteria for LVH alone without resting ST-T changes.
- An exercise ECG test without ST-segment deviation argues against the presence of flow-limiting CAD.

Bundle Branch Block/Ventricular Pacing

- The repolarization abnormalities associated with left bundle branch block (LBBB) or ventricular pacing accentuate with exercise, making the exercise ECG test unreliable in the diagnosis of CAD. As such, patients with these findings on their resting ECG should have stress testing in combination with myocardial imaging.
- Transient development of LBBB during exercise is associated with higher incidence of major adverse cardiovascular events and death.
- Resting right bundle branch block (RBBB) does not interfere with interpretation of the exercise ECG, although the pre-existing ST-segment deviation in the anterior precordial leads (V2–V3) may be accentuated by exercise.
- Exercise-induced RBBB is usually rate-dependent and not related to the presence of CAD.

Ventricular Pre-Excitation/Wolff-Parkinson-White (WPW) Pattern/Syndrome

- Exercise testing is commonly used in patients with ventricular pre-excitation syndromes to help stratify risk of developing rapid ventricular response during atrial arrhythmias by evaluating the effect of exercise and increased heart rate (HR) on anomalous atrioventricular (AV) conduction.
- Among patients where pre-excitation is not extinguished by exercise, significant ST-segment and T-wave abnormalities can occur (Figures 15.1 – 15.3), similar to patients with LVH with "strain pattern" or LBBB. Thus, these findings should not be interpreted as being indicative of myocardial ischemia.

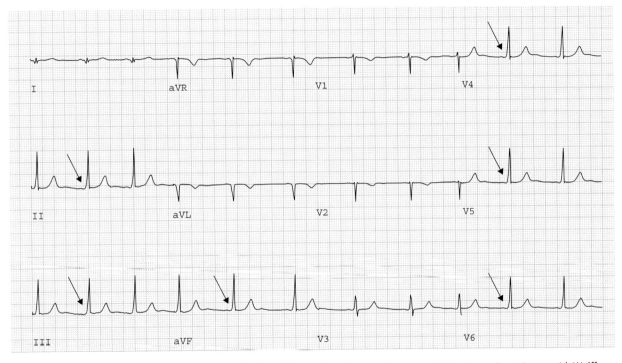

Figure 15.1 Resting ECG showing sinus rhythm with short PR interval and ventricular pre-excitation (arrow) consistent with Wolff-Parkinson-White Syndrome. ST segments at baseline are normal.

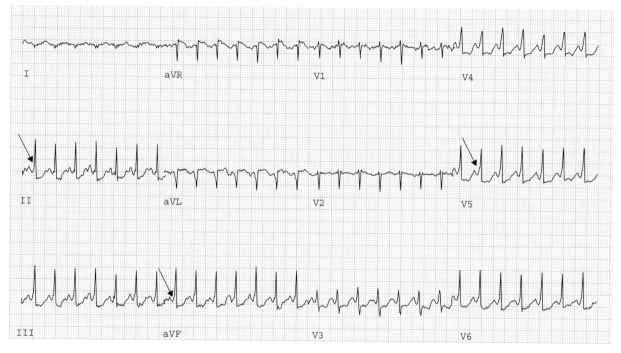

Figure 15.2 Peak stress ECG showing 1-2 mm horizontal ST depression consistent with an ischemic response. Ventricular pre-excitation persists (arrow). In this setting, persistent pre-excitation suggests the ST response is a false positive.

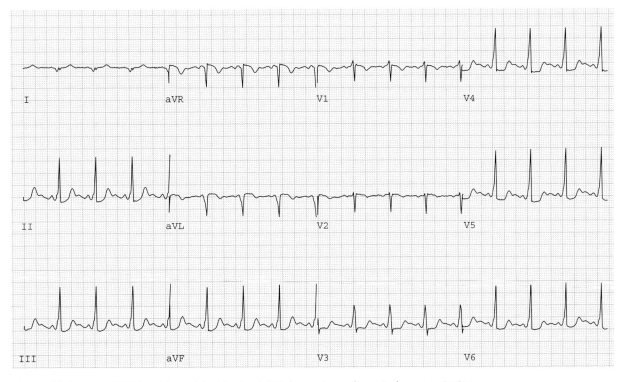

Figure 15.3 Recovery ECG showing persistent horizontal ST depression and ventricular pre-excitation.

Resting ST-Segment Depression

Similar to other conditions listed above that affect repolarization, ST-segment depression ≥0.5–1.0 mm on the resting ECG is associated with a higher incidence of false-positive exercise ECG test results.

Women

- Exercise ECG stress testing in women is hampered by a lower specificity of ST-segment changes for myocardial ischemia compared to men.
- Reasons for the lower predictive power of the stress ECG are not clearly defined, but may be due to a combination of a lower overall prevalence of CAD than men, a higher prevalence of non-obstructive CAD and microvascular disease, and higher incidence of false-positive exercise-induced ST segment depression.
- Patients with suspected false-positive stress ECG results should undergo testing with myocardial imaging, which comes at an increased cost and exposure to ionizing radiation if myocardial perfusion imaging (MPI) is used.
- A recent randomized, controlled trial evaluated women with intermediate pre-test probability of CAD with exercise stress ECG testing or exercise MPI and found that although the exercise ECG leads to more abnormal testing, and more follow-up testing, overall costs were lower and clinical outcomes were equivalent.

Hypokalemia

- Hypokalemia, common among patients receiving diuretics, may produce false-positive stress ECG results, especially in the presence of resting ST-segment abnormality.
- Use of diuretic therapy, without the presence of hypokalemia, is not sufficient to cause ST-segment depression.

Computer Processing

- Computer-aided processing of ECG waveforms can be used to help interpret the stress ECG and identify ischemic changes. However, such processing may exaggerate the ECG findings and tend to increase the rate of false-positive testing. To avoid this, it is recommended that interpreting physicians be provided with raw ECG data and any computer-aided processing be clearly labeled and separated from raw data.

Atrial Repolarization (T-a) Wave

- Atrial repolarization waves occur opposite in direction to P-waves and may extend into the ST-segment and T-wave.
- Exaggeration of atrial repolarization waves during exercise has been shown to be a cause of ST-segment depression that may mimic myocardial ischemia.
- Steeply down-sloping PR-segments, particularly when observed in the inferior ECG leads during exercise, may serve as a marker of this phenomenon.

False-Negative Exercise ECG Responses

Submaximal Exercise

- Submaximal exercise significantly reduces the sensitivity of the exercise ECG stress test to detect CAD.
- Exercise may be limited by several factors such as physical barriers to exercise, as with orthopedic or neurological disease, inability to negotiate the treadmill, medications that limit maximum HR, or claudication symptoms from peripheral arterial disease.
- Patients who have a submaximal effort test or in whom a submaximal effort is suspected in advance of testing should be considered for pharmacological stress imaging.

Beta-Adrenergic Blocking Agents

- Although individual beta-blockers vary in their specificity to affect cardiac beta receptors, the class in general exhibits negative chronotropic and inotropic effects, thereby reducing myocardial oxygen consumption for any given workload.
- Negative chronotropic effect may prevent subjects from reaching their target HR.
- Likewise, the maximum rate-pressure product may be reduced and subjects may not be able to reach an ischemic rate-pressure product. Patients with CAD therefore may be able to exercise for longer time without developing ischemic symptoms or ST-segment deviation, lowering the sensitivity of the test.
- However, data on the actual effect of beta-blockade on stress testing is lacking, with one cohort study of men undergoing exercise ECG testing for CAD showing no difference in test performance between patients taking and not taking beta-blockers.

Calcium Channel Blockers

- Calcium channel blockers have similar antianginal efficacy to beta-blockers, albeit through a different mechanism, by increasing coronary blood flow and reducing myocardial oxygen consumption. They have specific utility in reducing ischemic episodes in vasospastic angina.
- In studies of patients with established CAD and chronic angina undergoing exercise ECG stress testing, nifedipine has been shown to improve exercise duration and reduce ischemic ST-segment changes, potentially reducing the sensitivity of the test.

Nitrates

- Nitrates exert their anti-anginal effects by dilating large epicardial coronary vessels as well as smaller intra-myocardial vessels. Additionally, they can reduce diastolic filling pressure. The summation of these effects is to improve coronary blood flow, reduce coronary steal syndromes, and improve myocardial perfusion.
- With exercise MPI, nitrate therapy has been shown to reduce the severity and extent of nuclear scan ischemia without significant effect on HR response, BP, or double product.
- Nitrate therapy allows patients with established CAD and chronic angina to exercise longer without symptoms and delays the ischemic ST-segment response, reducing the sensitivity of exercise stress ECG testing. As with beta-blockers and calcium channel blockers, there are no guideline recommendations for the discontinuation of nitrates prior to testing.

L-arginine

- L-arginine is an alpha-amino acid and a precursor in the synthesis of nitric oxide.
- Administration of L-arginine has been shown to promote vasodilation and improve coronary microvascular blood flow.
- Although the effects on exercise stress ECG are not known, a small double-blind trial of patients on L-arginine for chronic stable angina showed an increase in exercise time, maximum workload, and a delay in ischemic ST-segment response.
- Due to a lack of data, however, there is no guideline recommendation for the discontinuation of L-arginine prior to stress testing.

Limited Extent or Severity of CAD

- A false-negative response may occur when the location of ischemia can be electrically silent relative to the body surface ECG. This finding is particularly true when ischemia is confined to the distribution of the left circumflex coronary artery.
- CAD of borderline angiographic significance (50–60% diameter stenosis), particularly when involving only a single epicardial coronary vessel, may not lead to ischemic ST-segment changes during the exercise ECG test.

Summary

- The exercise ECG stress test has reasonable sensitivity and specificity for the detection of ischemic heart disease, although false-positive and false-negative tests can and do occur.
- False-positive results typically occur in the setting of an abnormal resting ECG (LBBB, LVH with repolarization changes, ventricular pre-excitation, digitalis use, and hypokalemia with resting ST-segment changes).
- Right bundle branch block does not interfere with interpretation of exercise ECG, although pre-existing ST-segment deviation in the anterior precordial leads (V2–V3) may be accentuated by exercise.
- Women and patients with mitral valve disease also have higher rates of false-positive results.
- False-negative results can be seen in patients receiving anti-anginal drug therapy (beta-blockers, calcium channel blockers, nitrates), among patients who fail to reach their age-predicted HR, with submaximal exercise bouts, and with CAD involving only a single vessel or of borderline angiographic significance.
- Despite the increased possibility of a false-negative response with anti-anginal drug therapy, the risks of withholding therapy prior to stress testing is felt to be higher than the reduction in false-negative tests, and therefore no recommendations exist to stop these medications in advance of testing.
- Clinicians ordering an exercise ECG stress test should be aware of its limitations in certain settings and consider use concomitant myocardial imaging or alternative testing strategies to improve diagnostic performance when appropriate.

References

Ceremuzyński, L., Chamiec, T., and Herbaczyńska-Cedro, K. (1997). Effect of supplemental oral L-arginine on exercise capacity in patients with stable angina pectoris. *Am. J. Cardiol.* 80: 331–333.

Del Campo, J., Do, D., Umann, T. et al. (1996). Comparison of computerized and standard visual criteria of exercise ECG for diagnosis of coronary artery disease. *Ann. Noninvasive Electrocardiol.* 1: 430–442.

Egashira, K., Hirooka, Y., Kuga, T. et al. (1996). Effects of L-arginine supplementation on endothelium-dependent coronary vasodilation in patients with angina pectoris and normal coronary arteriograms. *Circulation* 94: 130–144.

Fletcher, G.F., Ades, P.A., Kligfield, P. et al., American Heart Association Exercise, Cardiac Rehabilitation, and Prevention Committee of the Council on Clinical Cardiology, Council on Nutrition, Physical Activity and Metabolism, Council on Cardiovascular and Stroke Nursing, and Council on Epidemiology and Prevention (2013). Exercise standards for testing and training: a scientific statement from the American Heart Association. *Circulation* 128: 873–934.

Gianrossi, R., Detrano, R., Mulvihill, D. et al. (1989). Exercise-induced ST depression in the diagnosis of coronary artery disease. A meta-analysis. *Circulation* 80: 87–98.

Gibbons, R.J., Balady, G.J., Bricker, J.T. et al., American College of Cardiology/American Heart Association Task Force on Practice Guidelines. Committee to Update the 1997 Exercise Testing Guidelines (2002). ACC/AHA 2002 guideline update for exercise testing: summary article. A report of the American College of Cardiology/American Heart Association Task Force on Practice Guidelines (Committee to Update the 1997 Exercise Testing Guidelines). *J. Am. Coll. Cardiol.* 40: 1531–1540. Erratum in: J Am Coll Cardiol 2006; 48: 1731.

Grady, T.A., Chiu, A.C., Snader, C.E. et al. (1998). Prognostic significance of exercise-induced left bundle-branch block. *JAMA* 279: 153–166.

Herbert, W.G., Dubach, P., Lehmann, K.G., and Froelicher, V.F. (1991). Effect of beta-blockade on the interpretation of the exercise ECG: ST level versus delta ST/HR index. *Am. Heart J.* 122 (4 Pt 1): 993–1000.

Mahmarian, J.J., Fenimore, N.L., Marks, G.F. et al. (1994). Transdermal nitroglycerin patch therapy reduces the extent of exercise-induced myocardial ischemia: results of a double-blind, placebo-controlled trial using quantitative thallium-201 tomography. *J. Am. Coll. Cardiol.* 24: 25–32.

Mieres, J.H., Gulati, M., Bairey Merz, N. et al., American Heart Association Cardiac Imaging Committee of the Council on Clinical Cardiology; Cardiovascular Imaging and Intervention Committee of the Council on Cardiovascular Radiology and Intervention (2014). Role of noninvasive testing in the clinical evaluation of women with suspected ischemic heart disease: a consensus statement from the American Heart Association. *Circulation* 130: 350–379. Erratum in: Circulation 2014; 130: c86.

Morise, A.P. and Diamond, G.A. (1995). Comparison of the sensitivity and specificity of exercise electrocardiography in biased and unbiased populations of men and women. *Am. Heart J.* 130: 741–747.

Rice, K.R., Gervino, E., Jarisch, W.R., and Stone, P.H. (1990). Effects of nifedipine on myocardial perfusion during exercise in chronic stable angina pectoris. *Am. J. Cardiol.* 65: 1097–1101.

Sapin, P.M., Koch, G., Blauwet, M.B. et al. (1991). Identification of false positive exercise tests with use of electrocardiographic criteria: a possible role for atrial repolarization waves. *J. Am. Coll. Cardiol.* 18: 127–135.

Shaw, L.J., Mieres, J.H., Hendel, R.H. et al. (2011). Comparative effectiveness of exercise electrocardiography with or without myocardial perfusion single photon emission computed tomography in women with suspected coronary artery disease: results from the What Is the Optimal Method for Ischemia Evaluation in Women (WOMEN) trial. *Circulation* 124: 1239–1249.

Sketch, M.H., Mooss, A.N., Butler, M.L. et al. (1981). Digoxin-induced positive exercise tests: their clinical and prognostic significance. *Am. J. Cardiol.* 48: 655–659.

Sundqvist, K., Atterhög, J.H., and Jogestrand, T. (1986). Effect of digoxin on the electrocardiogram at rest and during exercise in healthy subjects. *Am. J. Cardiol.* 57: 661–665.

16 Pediatric Exercise Testing

Thomas W. Rowland and Dennis A. Tighe

Introduction

The goal of clinical exercise testing in children is no different than in adults – examining the physiological and symptomatic responses to induced functional stress on the heart and lungs. However, a number of factors make such testing different in immature subjects, as compared to adults. Successful testing can be performed in youngsters as young as three to five years of age, but their differences from adults must be carefully considered when performing exercise stress tests.

The principal differences that separate pediatric from adult exercise testing which will be reviewed in this chapter are:

- The indications for exercise testing in children are more diverse than those in adults, in whom the principal focus often is on assessment of coronary artery insufficiency.

Pocket Guide to Stress Testing, Second Edition. Edited by Dennis A. Tighe and Bryon A. Gentile.
© 2020 John Wiley & Sons Ltd. Published 2020 by John Wiley & Sons Ltd.

- The wide range of size of subjects during the pediatric years necessitates a more flexible approach to selecting an appropriate testing protocol. In some situations (i.e. measurement of maximal oxygen uptake) such differences in body size can also influence selection of proper equipment.
- Children are emotionally immature compared to adults and need special attention, encouragement, and support as well as proper safety precautions during testing.

Indications for Exercise Testing of Children

- Coronary artery disease is rare in children, thus indications for exercise testing encompass a broader range of clinical situations than testing in adults.
- Testing of children is valuable in assessing more than simply cardiovascular function. Pediatric exercise testing has been utilized in the evaluation of a wide range of endocrine, musculoskeletal, metabolic, gastrointestinal, and pulmonary disorders.

Assessing Cardiopulmonary Functional Capacity

- Cardiac functional reserve can be evaluated by exercise endurance time, estimation of cardiac output (Q), or measurement of oxygen uptake (metabolic testing).
- This information may be useful in guiding therapeutic interventions for patients with cardiac disease.
- Estimation of pulmonary function during exercise testing is helpful in the care of children with chronic lung disease, such as cystic fibrosis.

Identifying Myocardial Ischemia

- While coronary insufficiency from atherosclerotic vascular disease is seldom a consideration, other causes of myocardial ischemia can be evaluated by exercise testing.
- Patients with congenital aortic stenosis often produce ischemic ST-segment changes on the ECG during exercise when the left ventricular (LV) outflow tract gradient is significant (typically >50 mmHg). Thus, exercise testing of these individuals can be useful in determining the need for intervention (surgery or balloon valvuloplasty).
- Other conditions in children which may manifest ischemic changes with exercise include Kawasaki disease, an inflammatory vasculitis that produces coronary artery aneurysms, and congenital hypoplasia or anomalous origins of coronary arteries.

Management of Young Athletes

- Several issues surrounding possible risk of training and competition in young athletes can be examined by exercise testing.
- Whether an elevated blood pressure (BP) response to exercise poses a risk for athletes is not clear; and if so, what level of BP should create concern? Excessive BP rise during exercise testing (systolic blood pressure (SBP) >240 mmHg) may signal a need for drug treatment.
- Great concern exists over athletes who experience syncope, chest pain, or dizziness during competition. While these symptoms may indicate presence of a serious underlying cardiac abnormality (i.e. hypertrophic cardiomyopathy, arrhythmogenic right ventricular dysplasia, anomalous origin of a coronary artery, ventricular arrhythmias), they most often are reflections of more benign, treatable conditions (dehydration, hyperthermia). Exercise testing is helpful in identifying the etiology of these symptoms.

Assessing Cardiac Rhythm and Rate

- Exercise testing can be used as a provocative technique for arrhythmias in children in the same manner as it is for adults.
- Exercise testing is particularly helpful in certain pediatric conduction system disturbances.
- In children with congenital complete heart block, for example, sinus node response to exercise is normal, but the rise in ventricular rate is dampened. It is not unusual for the ventricular rate to increase from a resting value of 45 bpm to a peak rate of only 60–80 bpm. The degree of ventricular rate response to exercise may provide information regarding the child's functional exercise capacity. This information may be important in timing of pacemaker implantation.
- Similar issues regarding heart rate (HR) response to exercise may be important in those children who demonstrate chronotropic incompetence after certain types of cardiac surgery.
- Exercise testing can be helpful in provoking arrhythmias, uncovering potentially diagnostic ECG abnormalities, and assessing response to therapy in certain cases of suspected tachyarrhythmias including:
  - Catecholaminergic polymorphic ventricular tachycardia (VT): exercise testing is the most reliable method to establish the diagnosis.
  - Arrhythmogenic right ventricular dysplasia: exercise may induce the typical monomorphic VT with left bundle branch block (LBBB)-pattern.
  - Congenital long QT-syndrome: diagnostic ECG abnormalities may be provoked and the response to beta-blocker therapy can be assessed.
  - Brugada syndrome: among patients with a type-1 pattern at rest, exercise may induce changes in the right precordial ST-segments that can aid in making a more firm diagnosis.
  - Exercise-induced supraventricular tachycardia (SVT): exercise testing may helpful in assessing SVTs that occur with exertion; in general, however, exercise testing is of limited utility in patients with SVT.

– Manifest Wolff-Parkinson-White (WPW) pattern: exercise testing can be used to assess the refractory period of an accessory pathway.

Evaluating Exercise-Induced Asthma

- The most common cause of chest pain during exercise in children is exercise-induced asthma.
- Assessment of children for exercise-induced asthma is one of the most common indications for exercise testing in the pediatric population.
- Children with this complaint can be evaluated by measurement of peak expiratory flow rates and other spirometric indices before and after exercise testing.
- In the typical child with wheezing, cough, and/or shortness of breath following exercise, such testing is not always necessary to make this diagnosis. However, formal laboratory exercise testing can be useful in examining the effects of therapy, identifying the cause in questionable cases, and distinguishing exercise-induced asthma from competitive breathlessness in athletes.

Assessing Physical Fitness

- Complaints of easy fatigability with exercise are common in children and adolescents.
- Assessment of exercise tolerance during treadmill or cycle testing can be a valuable means of establishing the validity of this concern as well as providing guidance for evaluation and management.
- Measurement of maximal/peak oxygen uptake (VO_{2max}) gives a numerical indicator of fitness; treadmill endurance time also provides a reasonable estimate.
- Body composition (i.e. adiposity) can have important influence influencing on these parameters.

Following the Course of Chronic Disease

- The ability of an individual to exercise depends not only on cardiac and pulmonary function but also on the contribution of musculoskeletal, hematologic, metabolic, and psychological factors.
- The natural course and response to therapy of diseases involving these systems (i.e. muscular dystrophy, sickle cell anemia) can be assessed through exercise testing.

Assessment of Rehabilitation Programs

- Children with chronic lung and heart diseases are often involved in exercise rehabilitation programs.
- Exercise testing is important in assessing the progress of these patients as well as identifying certain risk factors (arrhythmias, myocardial ischemia).

Children's Responses to Exercise

- A number of physiological differences exist in the responses of children to exercise compared with adults.
- It is important that staff performing testing of children be aware of such features, as these may influence the interpretation of test results.

Heart Rate

- The most obvious feature of the cardiovascular response to exercise in children is their higher HR.
- Resting and submaximal exercise HR progressively declines during the pediatric years and into young adulthood. For instance, a 10-year-old subject's HR at rest and at a given treadmill work load will be approximately 10–20 bpm higher as compared to a 25-year-old patient.

- Maximal HR as well is greater in children than adults.
- Contrary to the trend observed in adults, peak HR does not decrease with age during the childhood years.
- Therefore, formulas such as 220 – age to estimate peak HR are not appropriate for use in the pediatric age group.
- The actual peak HR depends on the particular exercise testing protocol being utilized.
- In general, maximal HR averages approximately 200 bpm during treadmill testing and 195 bpm for cycle testing for both healthy boys and girls across the pediatric years.
- Maximal exercise HR does begin to decline during the late teens.
- It is important to recognize the existence of a wide inter-individual variability in maximal exercise HR in children. Within any group of 12-year-old children, for example, maximal HR during treadmill testing may range from 190 to 215 bpm.
- Therefore, while peak HR during an exercise test is of some use in estimating whether a true maximal effort was provided, subjective observation of the patient for evidence of exhaustion can often be more accurate.

Blood Pressure

- Resting, submaximal, and maximal SBP responses progressively increase during the childhood and adolescent years.
- A typical maximal SBP in a healthy child with a body surface area (BSA) of $1.25 \, m^2$ is 140 mmHg, while that of the child with a BSA of $1.75 \, m^2$ is 160 mmHg.

Endurance Time

- Exercise endurance time is often used as an indicator of cardiovascular or aerobic fitness.
- During the childhood years, duration of exercise during laboratory testing is strongly influenced by age.

- Studies of healthy subjects undergoing treadmill testing with the Bruce protocol indicate that average endurance time increases from 9 minutes at ages 6–7 years to 12 minutes at age 12.
- Endurance times tend to be somewhat longer in boys than girls. Males increase their endurance time to an average peak of 13–14 minutes from ages 16–18, after which times begin to decline.
- Females peak at age 12, with an average duration of 12 minutes before exhibiting a progressive decrease in endurance.

Electrocardiographic Changes

- In general, responses of the ECG to exercise (shortened PR- and QT-intervals, increased P-wave voltage) are similar in children and adults.
- An increase in R-wave voltage with exercise is frequently observed in normal healthy children.
- ST-segment changes which have been interpreted as indicative of ischemia in adults, have also been used as criteria in pediatric patients.
- However, the validity of these alterations as signs of coronary insufficiency in children is uncertain.

Other Factors

- A number of other physiological features distinguish children from adults during exercise testing. While these factors may not have a direct bearing on interpretation of test results, staff performing exercise testing on children should be aware of these differences.
  - Children sweat less than adults during exercise, related to a diminished sweat output per gland. As a result, maximal testing will often produce little or no sweat in a child compared to the profusely sweating adult.

- For reasons that are not clear, children recover physiologically from intense bouts of exercise more rapidly than do adult subjects.
- During submaximal exercise, children demonstrate lower energy economy than adults, requiring a greater energy expenditure (oxygen uptake) per body mass than mature individuals.
- Children have less anaerobic capacity relative to their body mass than adults and are therefore less capable of short-burst, high-intensity exercise.

Performing Exercise Testing in Children

- Obtaining accurate information from exercise testing is dependent on a properly conducted test.
- The approach to testing of children is no different from that in adults: choosing the best testing modality, using an appropriate testing protocol, and assuring accurate monitoring of physiological variables.

Testing Modality

- Clinical testing of children has been conducted with both cycle ergometer and treadmill.
- Both methods have particular advantages and disadvantages which dictate choice for a given test.
- A major factor in this decision, however, is the testing experience by the staff in a given laboratory.
- In the United States, a treadmill is more often used as the modality for exercise testing than is a cycle ergometer.

Cycle Testing

- Compared to treadmill, the cycle is cheaper, quieter, safer, and less intimidating to test subjects. The latter two are particularly important issues for younger children. Moreover, most children have previous experience with cycling.
- Certain physiological measurements, particularly BP, are more accurately measured during exercise on the cycle.
- Some significant disadvantages of the cycle for clinical testing are recognized, particularly for young children, including:
  - A proper test requires that children cycle at a constant pedaling rate (usually 50–60 rpm), often a difficult task for young (age <6 years), obese, or poorly fit subjects.
  - Maximal effort is entirely volitional, which may result in an inadequate exercise effort in these same groups of patients.
- As a result, performance on cycle testing may be limited by local muscle fatigue rather than the limits of cardiovascular function.
- The effect of local muscle fatigue may be greater among children, who have a relatively under-developed knee extensor muscle mass as compared to adults.

Treadmill Testing

- Treadmills are louder, more expensive, less portable, and more intimidating to children.
- However, the treadmill requires only that the child maintain the pace of the belt, and peak effort may be greater than on the cycle. For this reason, treadmill testing is generally preferred for young children.
- With small patients, increased risk of injury from falling on the treadmill requires greater diligence from the testing staff.

- Treadmill testing protocols produce a 10–20% greater stress on the cardiovascular system at maximal exercise in children as well as adults.
- Submaximal measurements such as BP are more difficult to obtain because of noise and patient movement.
- Therefore, patients in whom BP measurements are particularly important (i.e. following coarctation repair) may be best tested on the cycle ergometer. Also, for some children with musculoskeletal abnormalities, walking on the treadmill may be difficult.

Testing Protocols

- Exercise testing of children involves a wide range of patient size and fitness, from the obese four-year-old with complete heart block to the 16-year-old competitive cross-country runner with complaints of chest pain during competition.
- The choice of protocol will depend on the purpose of the test and the characteristics of the patient. Consequently, no single standard exercise testing protocol has been adopted for children.
- To ensure that adequate information is derived from the stress test, an exercise protocol should be chosen to have the subject achieve their limit of tolerance in 10 ± 2 minutes.
- Most clinical laboratories use the Bruce treadmill protocol or its modification (see Chapter 5) for pediatric subjects, principally because of its familiarity from experience in testing adults.
- There are certain disadvantages of the Bruce protocol for use in children, which include:
  - Work increments between successive stages may be too great or too long for young subjects; some subjects may tend to quit during the first minute of a new stage.
  - For very fit subjects, the first four stages of the protocol may be too slow, leading to boredom.
  - Work increments are unequal.
    The protocol changes speed and slope at the same time, making adaptation more difficult for unfit subjects.

– Most exercise is performed at relatively steep slopes.
– Highly fit subjects (such as high school runners) have to wait 12 minutes before even breaking into a run (and then at a high slope).
• For these reasons, other protocols have been utilized in the pediatric population.

Treadmill Protocols

• *Bruce protocol:* The Bruce protocol, despite its recognized limitations, does offer certain advantages for clinical testing of children, including:
  – Relates endurance to published norms as well as maximal oxygen uptake.
  – Compares endurance longitudinally as well as between individuals.
  – Has widespread laboratory familiarity.
• *Balke protocols:* The Balke protocol and its modifications ("modified protocols") involve a constant treadmill speed with increases in slope. Balke protocols are usually utilized in pediatric research and less often in the clinical exercise testing laboratory.
  – Modified Balke protocols offer the advantage of producing a maximal treadmill effort at a comfortable speed and relatively low incline.
  – The stages are uniform, and only one variable (slope) is changed during the test. The treadmill incline is typically increased by 2–2.5% every two to three minutes. The speed of the treadmill is selected based on the child's fitness.
  – Walking protocols are utilized for young (less than eight to nine years), obese, or poorly fit subjects, with a constant speed of 2.75–3.5 mph.
  – Older and more fit patients perform a running protocol with speeds of 5.0–5.75 mph. Walking tests in this group of subjects usually results in an overly-long test at a steep incline.
  – An example of a modified Balke treadmill protocol for children and adolescents is outlined in Table 16.1. Using this protocol, test duration is usually 10–12 minutes, regardless of fitness level.

Table 16.1 Modified Balke treadmill protocol.

Subject	Speed (mph)	Initial grade (%)	Increment (%)	Stage duration (min)
Poorly fit	3.0	6	2	2
Sedentary	3.25–3.5	6	2	2
Active	5.0	0	2.5	2
Athlete	5.25–5.5	0	2.5	2

Cycle Protocols

- Several cycle exercise protocols have been used for testing children.
- These protocols typically involve a pedaling rate of 50–60 rpm and vary in stage duration (usually one to three minutes), initial work load, and load increments according to body size.
- The most commonly used cycle protocols in pediatric patients have been the James, Godfrey, and McMaster protocols. The details of each are outlined in Table 16.2.

Alternative Protocols

- For children unable to perform a standard exercise test, alternative methods to assess cardiac function are available:
  - Six-minute walk test: may be applicable to children with moderate to severe exercise impairment. The primary outcome is the total distance walked in six minutes.

Table 16.2 Cycle ergometer protocols for children.

	Rate (rpm)	Body measure	Initial load	Increment	Stage duration (min)
McMaster	50	Height (cm)	Watts	Watts	
		<120	12.5	12.5	2
		120–140	12.5	25	2
		140–160	25	25	2
		>160	25	50 (male)	2
				25 (female)	2
James	60–70	Surface area (m^2)	(kg m/min)	(kg m/min)	
		<1.0	200	100	3
		1.0–1.2	200	200	3
		>1.2	200	300	3
Godfrey	60	Height (cm)	Watts	Watts	
		<120	10	10	1
		120–150	15	15	1
		>150	20	20	1

– Pharmacological stress testing (see Chapter 8): applicable when exercise testing is unsuitable or impractical. Insertion of an IV catheter to administer the pharmacological agent is required. Concomitant myocardial imaging with perfusion agents or echocardiography is necessary.

Special Considerations for Testing Children

Children are both physically and emotionally immature. Consequently, to achieve a satisfactory test, the testing staff must devote more time and attention to preventing anxiety and any lack of motivation among pediatric patients. That is, the child cannot be viewed simply as a "small adult." Several issues are particularly important

Staff Support

- There is no more essential contributor to a successful exercise test in children than a warm, enthusiastic, encouraging staff experienced in working with young patients.
- Pediatric subjects are often intimidated by the array of equipment in the testing laboratory and concern over being "tested." This anxiety is counterproductive in the goal to produce a maximal exercise test.
- A relaxed testing atmosphere with a friendly, thorough explanation to the child of the nature of the test is important in allaying test anxiety.
- The staff should explain that the test is not painful, but he or she will be asked to "work hard."
- Describing the test in terms of real-life experiences may be helpful ("at the end of the test it will feel like you're walking up a steep hill").
- Whether or not the child's parents or guardians should be allowed in the testing laboratory is controversial.
- Some feel that their presence may distract the child, or that adult-child conflicts may be reflected in the child's lack of desire to satisfy testing goals.

- Others consider the parent/guardian presence as a strong motivating factor for the child.
- If the parent or guardian is allowed in the room, it is often best if he/she is out of the child's line of sight.

Safety

- Since exercise testing by its nature poses some risks, it is important that the safety of the child be assured; the need for the information to be obtained by exercise testing should be carefully weighed against its potential risks. In general, stress testing in children has been shown to be very safe and carry an extremely low risk of serious complications (less than 0.035%).
- Absolute contraindications to exercise testing in children testing are similar to those encountered in adults (see Chapter 4) and include: active or acute myocardial or pericardial inflammatory disease, severe outflow tract obstruction, decompensated HF, and severe, uncontrolled arrhythmias.
- Relative risks to performing exercise stress testing in pediatric patients are recognized (Table 16.3).
- General indications to terminate an exercise test in children are similar to adult testing (see Chapter 5):
  - When diagnostic findings have been established or a pre-determined end-point has been reached.
  - When monitoring equipment fails.
  - When signs or symptoms indicate a potential hazard that may result in injury.
- The child who is exercising on a treadmill, particularly a very young or uncoordinated patient, needs to be protected against falling. A staff member must stand at the child's side and serve as a "spotter."
- Children often do not communicate well with staff during exercise testing, so those conducting the test must pay special attention to ensure the well-being of the patient and the proper functioning of equipment.
- Side handrails at an appropriate height for the child are important in the pediatric testing laboratory (although most laboratories insist on the subject using the handrails but only for momentary support).
- Written informed consent for the test should be obtained from a parent or guardian of the child prior to testing. Verbal assent should be obtained from the child if over the age of seven or eight years.

Table 16.3 Relative risks for stress testing.

Lower risk

- Symptoms during exercise in an otherwise healthy child with a normal cardiac examination and ECG.
- Exercise-induced bronchospasm studies in the absence of severe resting airways obstruction.
- Asymptomatic patients undergoing evaluation for possible long-QTc syndrome.
- Asymptomatic ventricular ectopy with a structurally normal heart.
- Unrepaired or residual congenital cardiac lesions and asymptomatic at rest, including:
  - Left to right shunts.
  - Obstructive right heart lesions without severe resting obstruction.
  - Obstructive left heart lesions without severe resting obstruction.
  - Regurgitant lesions regardless of severity.
- Routine follow-up of asymptomatic patients at risk for myocardial ischemia, including:
  - Kawasaki disease without giant aneurysms or known coronary stenosis.
  - After repair of anomalous left coronary artery.
  - After arterial switch procedure.
- Routine monitoring in cardiac transplant patients not currently experiencing rejection.
- Presence of palliated cardiac lesions without uncompensated heart failure (HF), arrhythmia, or extreme cyanosis.
- History of hemodynamically stable supraventricular tachycardia (SVT).
- Stable dilated cardiomyopathy without uncompensated HF or documented arrhythmia.

Higher risk

- Presence of pulmonary hypertension.
- Documented long-QTc syndrome.
- Dilated/restrictive cardiomyopathy with HF or arrhythmia.

(Continued)

Table 16.3 (Continued)

- History of a hemodynamically unstable arrhythmia.
- Hypertrophic cardiomyopathy with any of the following features:
  - Symptoms.
  - Greater than mild LV outflow tract obstruction.
  - Documented arrhythmia.
- Greater than moderate airways obstruction on baseline pulmonary function tests.
- Marfan's syndrome and activity-related chest pain where a non-cardiac cause of chest pain is suspected.
- Suspected myocardial ischemia with exertion.
- Routine testing of patients with Marfan's syndrome.
- Unexplained syncope with exercise.

Source: Adapted with permission from: Paridon et al. (2006).

Summary

- The basic tenets of clinical exercise testing are the same in adults and children.
- Certain aspects unique to the testing of children should be appreciated:
  - The immaturity of children requires particular attention to safety and a great deal of staff support and encouragement.
  - Physiologic norms are different in children (i.e. higher maximal HRs, lower BP).
  - The wide range of size of pediatric subjects requires adaptability when selecting testing protocols.
  - Indications for exercise testing are broader in children.

References

Chang, R.R., Gurvitz, M., Rodriguez, S. et al. (2006). Current practice of exercise stress testing among pediatric cardiology and pulmonology centers in the United States. *Pediatr. Cardiol.* 27: 110–116.

Cifra, B., Dragulescu, A., Border, W.L., and Mertens, L. (2015). Stress echocardiography in paediatric cardiology. *Eur. Heart J. Cardiovasc. Imaging* 16: 1051–1059.

Massin, M.M. (2014). The role of exercise testing in pediatric cardiology. *Arch. Cardiovasc. Dis.* 107: 319–327.

Paridon, S.M., Alpert, B.S., Boas, S.R. et al., American Heart Association Council on Cardiovascular Disease in the Young, Committee on Atherosclerosis, Hypertension, and Obesity in Youth (2006). Clinical stress testing in the pediatric age group: a statement from the American Heart Association Council on Cardiovascular Disease in the Young, Committee on Atherosclerosis, Hypertension, and Obesity in Youth. *Circulation* 113: 1905–1920.

Takken, T., Bongers, B.C., van Brussel, M. et al. (2017). Cardiopulmonary exercise testing in pediatrics. *Ann. Am. Thorac. Soc.* 14: S123–S128.

Washington, R.L., Bricker, J.T., Alpert, B.S. et al. (1994). Guidelines for exercise testing in the pediatric age group. From the Committee on Atherosclerosis and Hypertension in Children, Council on Cardiovascular Disease in the Young, the American Heart Association. *Circulation* 90: 2166–2179.

17 Follow-up Care and Management

Dennis A. Tighe

Introduction

The exercise test offers important diagnostic and prognostic information. The information acquired from the patient's clinical history and physical examination must be integrated with data obtained from the ECG response to stress, the stress-induced hemodynamic responses, and the results of myocardial imaging (if performed) in order to direct and optimize therapy for the individual patient. Abundant literature is available to guide the clinician in this task. This chapter will review the information available from the stress test, which can provide prognostic implications and guide further therapy. Prognostic implications of cardiac stress testing among patients following recent acute coronary syndromes are discussed in Chapter 10.

Pocket Guide to Stress Testing, Second Edition. Edited by Dennis A. Tighe and Bryon A. Gentile.
© 2020 John Wiley & Sons Ltd. Published 2020 by John Wiley & Sons Ltd.

General Principles and Goals of Exercise Stress Testing

- The major goals of optimal cardiac stress testing include diagnosis of coronary artery disease (CAD), assessment of the functional status of the heart (functional capacity), and prediction of future cardiac events (prognosis).
- It is well recognized that coronary artery anatomy demonstrated by coronary angiography does not necessarily correlate with the functional significance of visualized stenotic lesions and the functional status of the heart.
- Exercise testing results should always be interpreted within the context of prevalence of disease within the population being evaluated (Bayes' theorem – see Chapter 11), the nature of the patient's symptoms, potential reasons for false-positive or false-negative results (Chapter 15), and the adequacy of the myocardial workload achieved.
- Patients should undergo exercise ECG stress testing rather than pharmacological testing whenever possible as the maximal diagnostic and prognostic information is obtained when the patient exercises as opposed to receiving infusion of a pharmacological agent.
- Myocardial imaging should be used to supplement standard exercise ECG testing in appropriate situations (see Chapters 6, 7, and 11).
- The vast majority of patients included in published studies of exercise testing have been men, although recent investigations have focused on the diagnostic and prognostic power of the exercise ECG test in women. Women do exhibit a higher incidence of false-positive studies likely due to lower CAD prevalence and test referral bias.
- Patients identified as being at high-risk for future atherosclerotic cardiovascular events from the results of stress testing should have their medical therapy intensified and, in most cases, be referred for coronary angiography.

Large Scale Studies Assessing Predictive Implications of Exercise ECG Stress Testing

- A number of studies have been published that assess the ability of the exercise ECG stress test to offer prognostic information.
- Despite discordant results regarding the prognostic implications of individual exercise test variables and the heterogeneity of the populations studied (known CAD versus suspected CAD; symptomatic versus asymptomatic patients), these studies consistently reveal that when a combination of abnormal stress-induced variables exist, significant prognostic information is provided.
- Based upon the presence or absence of these abnormal stress-induced variables, patients with a high or low risk of future cardiac events can be identified. In addition, most studies have shown that the combination of clinical and exercise-induced variables is superior to either used in isolation.

Individual Studies

Ellestad and Wan

- *Ellestad and Wan* demonstrated in a population of 2700 predominantly male subjects that a positive maximal exercise ECG stress test, defined as ≥1.5 mm of ST-segment depression, predicted the incidence of new coronary events (myocardial infarction [MI], death, progressive angina) to be 9.5% per year compared to 1.7% per year among those with a negative ECG response to maximal stress.
  - Early onset ischemia occurring at a low exercise workload (≤4 METs) was associated with a coronary event rate of 15% per year.
  - Ischemia occurring at a relatively high level of exercise (≥8 METs) was associated with a coronary event rate of 4% per year.

- Subjects with a normal ST-segment response to exercise, but inadequate chronotropic response compared to age and sex-matched controls, had an incidence of coronary events similar to those with ≥1.5 mm of ST-segment depression.
- Interestingly, these investigators found no relationship between either age or the magnitude of ST-segment depression and the incidence of future coronary events.
- *Limitations:* The limitations of this study include the heterogeneous nature of subjects studied (previous MI, symptomatic angina, and normal subjects) and a lack of stratification based upon treatment status.

Coronary Artery Surgery Study (CASS)

- *Coronary Artery Surgery Study* (CASS) investigators evaluated 4083 patients with suspected or proven CAD without previous cardiac surgery referred for exercise ECG stress testing within one month of coronary angiography.
  - Thirty total variables were analyzed: 18 clinical or historical; 7 from the exercise test; and 5 obtained at cardiac catheterization.
  - The duration of exercise and the ST-segment response to exercise were the variables obtained from exercise testing which predicted future events.
  - A low-risk group with an annual mortality of ≤1% was characterized by the ability to exercise to at least Stage III of the Bruce protocol with <1 mm of ST-segment depression.
  - A high-risk group with an annual mortality of ≥5% was identified by the inability to complete Stage I of the Bruce protocol, along with ≥1 mm of ST-segment depression.
  - Among the subgroup of patients with triple-vessel CAD, the probability of survival at four years was only 53% among those unable to complete Stage 1/2 (2 METs) as compared to 100% among those able to exercise into Stage V of the Bruce protocol.

- In addition to exercise variables, clinical variables such as presence of heart failure (HF) at rest, prior MI, cardiac enlargement; and catheterization variables such as left ventricular (LV) contraction pattern and number of diseased vessels were important predictors of survival.
- This study suggested that the prognosis of patients with CAD is dependent not only upon coronary anatomy, but more importantly upon the functional status of the LV and the exercise capacity.
- *Limitations:* The main limitation of this study is that the data is applicable only to symptomatic patients with proven or suspected CAD referred for coronary angiography and left ventriculography. In addition, the sex of the subjects studied was not specified, but most likely the vast majority of patients were men.

Mark and colleagues from Duke University

- *Mark and colleagues from Duke University* have derived a quantitative exercise treadmill score for predicting prognosis among those referred for exercise ECG testing.
  - An initial cohort consisted of symptomatic inpatients who had cardiac catheterization; 70% were men, and all patients had a Bruce protocol treadmill exercise ECG stress test within six weeks of coronary angiography.
  - Three independent prognostic treadmill (exercise) variables were identified:
    1) Total Bruce protocol exercise time in minutes
    2) Maximum ST-segment deviation (horizontal or downsloping ST-segment depression or ST-segment elevation in leads without q-waves or in lead aVR) in mm
    3) Treadmill angina index (defined as 0 = no angina; 1 = non-limiting typical angina; 2 = limiting angina which caused test termination)
  - The investigators found that a treadmill score that incorporated these exercise-related variables offered important prognostic information independent of the clinical and angiographic data. The Duke treadmill exercise score (DTS) was calculated as:

$$DTS = Exercise\ time - (5 \times ST - segment\ deviation) - (4 \times Treadmill\ angina\ index)$$

- The risk categories based upon the calculated exercise treadmill score were identified as:
    1) *High-risk:* A treadmill score <−10, associated with a five-year survival rate of 72%.
    2) *Moderate-risk:* A treadmill score of −10 to +4, associated with a five-year survival rate of 91%
    3) *Low-risk:* A treadmill score ≥+5, associated with a five-year survival rate of 97%.
- The corresponding cardiac event (MI or sudden death) rates were 63%, 86%, and 93%, respectively.
- The Duke investigators subsequently applied their exercise treadmill score to a group of 613 consecutive outpatients (67% male) with suspected CAD referred for exercise ECG stress testing. The investigators found that the treadmill score was a better indicator of prognosis than clinical data and was more useful among outpatients than among inpatients.
    1) *Low-risk:* A treadmill score ≥+5, associated with a four -year survival rate of 99%.
    2) *Moderate-risk:* A treadmill score between −10 and +4, associated with a four-year survival rate of 95%.
    3) *High-risk:* A treadmill score <−10, associated with a four-year survival rate of 79%.
- Subsequent examination of the coronary anatomy in relation to the DTS showed that as the risk classification by exercise testing worsened, the presence, severity, and extent of underlying CAD was greater; subjects with high-risk DTS had more extensive, often multi-vessel disease, whereas those classified as low-risk most often had no significant CAD or single-vessel disease.
- Implications: Identification of a large, low-risk group in whom prognosis is excellent and medical therapy is indicated as initial treatment. Stratification of patients into high- and intermediate-risk groups. In the high-risk group coronary angiography is warranted due to increased mortality risk. In the intermediate risk-group, repeat stress testing with myocardial imaging may help to further risk stratify these patients.

Seattle Heart Watch

- The Seattle Heart Watch Study investigators evaluated 3611 men and 547 women without clinical evidence of coronary heart disease who underwent symptom-limited, maximal Bruce protocol exercise ECG stress testing.
- Patients were separated into one of three groups:
  1) Asymptomatic healthy persons without clinical evidence of CAD.
  2) Atypical chest pain syndrome.
  3) Hypertension with normal ECG.
- Conventional risk factors for CAD (positive family history, hypertension, smoking, cholesterol level) and exercise test variables (workload less than Stage II, blunted HR response, chest pain with testing, and ST-segment depression) were assessed for each group.
- Patients were followed for the occurrence of cardiac events:
  - Among asymptomatic men, the combination of any single risk factor for CAD along with ≥2 exercise test variables identified 1% of healthy men with a 33-fold increased risk of a cardiac event.
  - Among asymptomatic men with no CAD risk factors, but with a "positive" ST-segment response to exercise, the likelihood of suffering a coronary event in the subsequent six years was "exceedingly small."
  - Among men with hypertension or atypical chest pain, the presence of one or more risk factors for CAD combined with at least one abnormal exercise test variable identified those with a "markedly lower" six-year survival rate without a cardiac event.
- *Implications:*
  - The interaction between conventional CAD risk factors and maximal exercise test variables for risk assessment among patients without clinically-evident CAD is important.

- ST-segment depression taken in isolation is not predictive of future cardiac events. Classification of ECG response to exercise by Bayesian analysis is necessary to obtain maximal predictive accuracy.
- Among men who are clinically free of CAD and without risk factors for CAD, exercise testing offered no apparent benefit to risk assessment.

- *Limitations:* The major limitations of this study were the inadequate number of women sampled to allow for firm conclusions to be drawn, and the small number of patients with diabetes in the sample population.

WOMEN (What Is the Optimal Method for Ischemia Evaluation in Women) Trial

- The WOMEN Trial investigators randomized 824 symptomatic women of low to intermediate risk who could perform a treadmill test to a strategy of standard exercise ECG stress testing versus exercise myocardial perfusion imaging.
  - The primary end-point of the trial was the two-year incidence of a composite of cardiac death, nonfatal MI, or hospital admission for ACS or HF.
  - About one-third of patients had ≥1 mm of exercise-induced ST-segment depression and about 12% had chest pain with exercise. One-third of the exercise ECG tests had indeterminate or abnormal ST-segments responses; only 9% of perfusion imaging results were abnormal.
  - At two years follow-up, event-free survival was similar in both testing arms.
- *Implications:* This randomized trial found no incremental benefit for an upfront imaging strategy among symptomatic women with an interpretable ECG and ability to perform an adequate exercise bout.
- *Limitations:* The major limitation of this trial was the lower than expected number of adverse cardiac events observed as the study population was of relatively low-risk; a longer follow-up period and larger study groups would be required to discern differences. In addition, criteria for an "indeterminate" test included 0.5–1.0 mm ST-segment changes, chest pain during exercise, and/or submaximal exercise tolerance while an "abnormal"

test was defined as ≥1 mm ST-segment changes; other "non-ECG responses" were not considered. Previous investigators have shown that a more integrative approach, such as using the DTS and other indices (chronotropic response, HR recovery, BP response), effectively stratifies women into diagnostic and prognostic categories.

Exercise ECG Parameters Associated with Prognosis

Duration of Exercise

- Numerous studies have consistently demonstrated that impaired exercise capacity is strongly associated with future coronary events and is an independent predictor of cardiac mortality.
- Despite the fact that exercise capacity is dependent upon physiologic variables other than cardiovascular functional status (pulmonary function, neurologic status, orthopedic impairment, metabolic abnormalities, and medication use), it is now established to be the most powerful predictor of future cardiac events and survival. Among men referred for exercise testing, each one-MET increase in exercise capacity conferred a 12% improvement in survival.
- Failure to complete Stage 2 of the Bruce Protocol or its equivalent (6–7 METs) identifies a group at higher risk of mortality regardless of the extent of underlying CAD or LV function.
- An exercise capacity exceeding 10 METs (at least Bruce Stage III) identifies a group with excellent survival regardless of the extent of underlying CAD or LV function.
- This point is illustrated by the data of Morris and colleagues as summarized in Table 17.1. Among subjects with ≥2 mm of ST-segment depression during exercise ECG testing, exercise capacity, expressed in MET levels achieved, is related to mortality.

Table 17.1 Survival among patients with ≥2 mm ST-segment depression during exercise ECG testing.

METs	% 6-yr survival with exercise-induced angina	% 6-yr survival without exercise-induced angina
≥13	100	97
≤10	94	87
≤7	80	64
≤5	44	60

Source: Adapted and reproduced with permission from: Morris et al. (1991).
METs, metabolic equivalents.

- For patients able to exercise to a level ≥ 10 METs, myocardial imaging (echocardiography or myocardial perfusion imaging) does not add significant prognostic value, often shows fails to show extensive evidence of myocardial ischemia, and rarely provides an indication for mechanical intervention.

Heart Rate Response to Exercise

- Chronotropic incompetence, the inability of the HR to increase commensurate with increased activity or demand, has been shown to be an *adverse* predictor of prognosis. It has been variably defined as failure to achieve 85% of the age-predicted maximum heart rate or a low chronotropic index.
- Earlier studies have shown that failure to attain a peak exercise HR during maximal exercise testing ≥120 beats/min (off beta-blockers) is correlated with an increased risk of cardiac events, regardless of the occurrence of ST-segment depression or the anatomical extent of CAD.

- In more recent cohorts of patients, chronotropic incompetence to exercise was shown to be predictive of increased mortality and cardiac events after adjusting for LV function and the severity of exercise-induced myocardial ischemia.

Time of Onset and Degree of ST-segment Depression

- Downsloping or horizontal ST-segment depression of ≥2 mm that occurs at a HR of ≤120 beats/min at a low work-load (≤6.5 METs) is strongly associated with more extensive CAD and poor prognosis.
- ST-segment depression occurring in ≥5 leads, lasting ≥5 minutes into the recovery phase is also correlated with poor prognosis and more extensive CAD.
- Although some studies indicate that ≥2 mm of horizontal or downsloping ST-segment depression is associated with adverse prognosis, other studies indicate that timing of onset and duration of ST-segment depression in association with an abnormal hemodynamic response to exercise are more important predictors of adverse prognosis than is mere depth of ST-segment depression alone.
- "Recovery only" ST-segment depression carries the same prognostic implications as does ST-segment depression which occurs during exercise.
- ST-segment depression that rapidly normalizes in the recovery period (within the first minute) in the absence of any high-risk features has been shown to be associated with low-risk and no apparent benefit from additional diagnostic testing.

Blood Pressure Response During or Following Exercise

- A *sustained* decrease of systolic blood pressure (SBP) of ≥10 mmHg or failure of the SBP to rise above 120 mmHg with progressive exercise is correlated with advanced (left main-stem or triple vessel) CAD and/or LV dysfunction.

- The SBP response to progressive exercise may be blunted or even slightly diminished in normal individuals as anaerobic threshold is reached and exceeded. In some normal subjects with a hyperadrenergic state, the BP may rise early in exercise, fall 10–20 mmHg as exercise continues, and then begin to rise again later in the exercise bout.
- Patients receiving antihypertensive medications may experience a decline in SBP with exercise.
- Among patients with asymptomatic, moderate or severe aortic stenosis, failure of SBP to rise or increase <20 mmHg with exercise has been associated with adverse prognosis and constitutes an indication for a valve intervention.

Exercise-Induced Angina Pectoris

- Cole and Ellstead, and Weiner and colleagues have demonstrated that exercise-induced angina pectoris, especially in the presence of an ischemic ST-segment response, is predictive of future coronary events and more extensive CAD.
- Among men, the presence of typical angina without ECG changes during exercise is also associated with future coronary events. The onset of angina at a low workload (≤4 METs) is associated with twice the coronary event rate as compared to angina occurring at a heavy workload (≥8 METs).

Ventricular Ectopy During or After Exercise

- Ventricular premature complexes (VPCs) can be observed in 7–20% of individuals during or after an exercise ECG stress test. Frequent ventricular ectopy during and/or after exercise (defined as seven or more VPCs per minute, ventricular bigeminy or trigeminy, ventricular couplets or triplets, ventricular tachycardia (VT), ventricular flutter, torsade de pointes, or ventricular fibrillation) is a much less common event (2–3%).
- Previous studies indicated that exercise-only VPCs were predictive of adverse cardiovascular outcomes. More contemporary data shows that ventricular ectopy occurring in recovery from exercise adversely affects prognosis while that occurring solely during exercise is of limited prognostic significance.

Post-exercise Heart Rate Recovery

- With progressive exercise, the observed increase in HR is due in part to a reduction in vagal tone. Immediately following an exercise bout, recovery of the HR is a function of vagal reactivation.
- Abnormal HR recovery has been variably defined:
  - With Bruce or modified Bruce treadmill exercise protocols: ≤12 beats/min reduction during the first minute after exercise with a 2-minute post-exercise cool-down period at 1.5 mph and 2.5% grade.
  - With an exercise echo procedure or when a cool-down period is not used: ≤18 beats/min during the first minute after abrupt cessation of exercise.
  - With various treadmill protocols: <22 beats/min or ≤42 beats/min at two minutes after exercise.
  - Some investigators have reported that late HR recovery, measured at five minutes after exercise, also provides prognostic information independent of early (one minute) HR recovery.
- Impaired recovery of the HR (most often determined at one minute after exercise), a phenomenon which occurs in 20–29% of patients, has been shown to be a predictor of all-cause mortality that is independent of exercise workload, the presence or absence of myocardial perfusion defects, changes in HR during exercise, or the angiographic extent of CAD.

Prognostic Value of Myocardial Imaging

- Myocardial imaging (perfusion imaging or echocardiography) should be used in conjunction with an exercise ECG stress test when baseline ECG abnormalities affecting repolarization exist, false negative or positive responses to exercise is anticipated, when equivocal or non-diagnostic results of standard stress ECG testing have been obtained, and with intermediate risk-DTS. Myocardial imaging is also required in conjunction with pharmacological stress testing.

- Due to its ability to localize ischemia and define its extent, myocardial imaging provides information beyond that available from the standard exercise ECG stress test. It should be used when it is clinically necessary to localize ischemia or assess myocardial viability.
- In general, unless a specific reason exists, the standard exercise ECG stress test should initially be performed without myocardial imaging.
- An equivocal or unexpected result with standard ECG stress testing or an intermediate-risk stress ECG test often necessitates repeating the test with myocardial imaging.

Myocardial Perfusion Imaging

- Normal myocardial perfusion imaging (MPI) with either exercise or pharmacological stress, even in the presence of angiographically significant CAD, indicates a favorable cardiac event-free prognosis. The annual rate of death or non-fatal MI is reported to be ≤1%, similar to that of the general population. Despite significant CAD by angiography, revascularization is unlikely to benefit this group of patients when guideline-directed medial therapy is used.
- When myocardial perfusion imaging is abnormal, several features correlate with functionally severe CAD and high risk of future cardiac events:
  - Multiple transient perfusion defects in more than one vascular territory.
  - Extensive ischemia/defects (involving ≥20% of the myocardium).
  - Large fixed defects.
  - Increased lung uptake of ^{201}Tl radiotracer (increased lung-heart ratio).
  - Stress-induced, transient LV cavity dilatation.
  - LVEF ≤45%.
- These findings generally indicate need for referral for cardiac catheterization.

- Numerous studies have shown that the extent of jeopardized myocardium, represented by the number and severity of myocardial segments showing transient perfusion defects, is an excellent predictor of future cardiac events and adverse prognosis.
- Patients with reversible (transient) myocardial ischemia have a higher incidence of future cardiac events than do patients with fixed defects. The cardiac event rate is exponentially related to the number of myocardial segments demonstrating transient perfusion defects.
- The prognostic information available from MPI should be considered in the context of baseline patient characteristics. Among patients with normal perfusion imaging, older patients, those with diabetes, those with known CAD and those unable to exercise (having pharmacological stress testing) have higher event rates compared to subjects without these characteristics.
- In patients undergoing pharmacological-MPI, the number and severity of reversible myocardial perfusion defects and the presence of transient LV cavity dilatation have been shown to be significant predictors of decreased cardiac event-free survival. Several studies have demonstrated that the inability to exercise is associated with a higher event rate even with normal perfusion imaging.
- ST-segment depression occurring with vasodilator infusion is correlated with more extensive CAD, as documented with perfusion imaging or coronary angiography.

Stress Echocardiography

The prognostic implications of stress echocardiography have been extensively studied.

Exercise Stress

- A normal baseline and post-exercise stress echocardiogram identifies patients with low short-term annual risk (0.4–0.9%) for cardiac events that is similar to that of a normal stress myocardial perfusion imaging scan.

- Several investigators have shown that the annual cardiac event rate increases as a function of the severity and extent of abnormal wall motion response to stress.
- Stress-induced wall motion abnormalities confer adverse risk for cardiac events; peak wall motion score index can risk stratify patients into low- (0.9%/year), intermediate- (3.1%/year), and high-risk (5.2%/year) groups for cardiac events.
- Transient ischemic dilatation of the LV cavity with stress has been shown to be a marker of severe and extensive angiographic CAD that is associated with a high risk of cardiac events.
- Patients who achieve a submaximal age-predicted maximal HR in the setting of a normal stress echocardiogram have a higher risk of cardiovascular events than those who attained a maximal level of stress.

Dobutamine Stress

- A negative dobutamine stress echocardiogram has been shown to be associated with a very low short-term risk for cardiac death (≤1% per year).
- In addition to baseline clinical risk factors, adverse cardiac outcomes with dobutamine stress echocardiography are correlated with the extent and severity and of wall motion abnormality at peak stress.
- Among patients with a normal dobutamine stress echocardiogram, adverse long-term outcomes have been associated with older age, male gender, diabetes mellitus, hypertension, history of CAD, increased pretest probability of CAD, and failure to achieve the target HR.

Summary

- Stress testing offers important diagnostic and prognostic information.
- The information available from the patient's history, physical examination, and clinical data must be integrated with the results of the stress test in order to direct and optimize therapy.

- Large scale studies assessing the prognostic value of exercise ECG testing consistently show that when a combination of abnormal stress-induced variables is present, the risk of a future cardiac event is significantly increased.
- Table 17.2 summarizes exercise ECG stress variables associated with advanced CAD and adverse long-term prognosis.
- Conversely, when none of these adverse prognostic signs are provoked during an adequate exercise ECG test, long-term event-free prognosis is excellent, regardless of the extent of CAD by angiography.
- Myocardial imaging techniques (when used in the proper clinical situation) offer diagnostic and prognostic information beyond that available from the exercise ECG portion of the stress test. A normal perfusion scan or echocardiogram following an adequate exercise workload portends an excellent prognosis.
- Evidence of multiple transient perfusion scan defects with myocardial perfusion imaging or multiple new wall motion abnormalities during stress echocardiography is associated with increased risk of multi-vessel CAD and adverse prognosis. Transient ischemic cavity dilation or reduced LVEF on myocardial imaging is associated with increased risk for adverse cardiac events.
- Patients with high-risk findings on stress testing/imaging should, in general, be referred for coronary angiography.

Table 17.2 Exercise ECG stress test variables associated with increased risk of multi-vessel CAD and adverse prognosis.

- Duration of symptom-limited exercise <6 METs
- Failure to attain a peak exercise HR ≥120 beats/min (off beta-blockers or non-dihydropyridine calcium channel blockers)
- Inability to increase SBP ≥20 mmHg over baseline, failure of peak SBP during exercise to exceed 120 mmHg, or an early or sustained decline in SBP (≥10 mmHg) with exercise.
- ST-segment depression of ≥2 mm at a low workload (≤4 METs) or that occurs in ≥5 ECG leads and lasts ≥5 minutes into the recovery phase.
- High-risk Duke treadmill score
- Exercise-induced chest pain

References

Alexander, K.P., Shaw, L.J., Shaw, L.K. et al. (1998). Value of exercise treadmill testing in women. *J. Am. Coll. Cardiol.* 32: 1657–1664. Erratum in: J. Am. Coll. Cardiol. 1999; 33: 289.

Barlow, P.A., Otahal, P., Schultz, M.G. et al. (2014). Low exercise blood pressure and risk of cardiovascular events and all-cause mortality: systematic review and meta-analysis. *Atherosclerosis* 237: 13–22.

Bourque, J.M., Holland, B.H., Watson, D.D., and Beller, G.A. (2009). Achieving an exercise workload of > or = 10 metabolic equivalents predicts a very low risk of inducible ischemia: does myocardial perfusion imaging have a role? *J. Am. Coll. Cardiol.* 54: 538–545.

Bruce, R.A., Hossack, K.F., DeRouen, T.A., and Hofer, V. (1983). Enhanced risk assessment for primary coronary heart disease events by maximal exercise testing: 10 years' experience of Seattle Heart Watch. *J. Am. Coll. Cardiol.* 2: 565–573.

Chaowalit, N., McCully, R.B., Callahan, M.J. et al. (2006). Outcomes after normal dobutamine stress echocardiography and predictors of adverse events: long-term follow-up of 3014 patients. *Eur. Heart J.* 27: 3039–3044.

Christman, M.P., Bittencourt, M.S., Hulten, E. et al. (2014). Yield of downstream tests after exercise treadmill testing: a prospective cohort study. *J. Am. Coll. Cardiol.* 63: 1264–1274.

Dewey, F.E., Kapoor, J.R., Williams, R.S. et al. (2008). Ventricular arrhythmias during clinical treadmill testing and prognosis. *Arch. Intern. Med.* 168: 225–234.

Elhendy, A., Mahoney, D.W., Khandheria, B.K. et al. (2003). Prognostic significance of impairment of heart rate response to exercise: impact of left ventricular function and myocardial ischemia. *J. Am. Coll. Cardiol.* 42: 823–830.

Ellestad, M.H. and Wan, M.K. (1975). Predictive implications of stress testing: follow-up of 2700 subjects after maximum treadmill stress testing. *Circulation* 51: 363–369.

Fine, N.M., Pellikka, P.A., Scott, C.G. et al. (2013). Characteristics and outcomes of patients who achieve high workload (≥10 metabolic equivalents) during treadmill exercise echocardiography. *Mayo Clin. Proc.* 88: 1408–1419.

Frolkis, J.P., Pothier, C.E., Blackstone, E.H., and Lauer, M.S. (2003). Frequent ventricular ectopy after exercise as a predictor of death. *N. Engl. J. Med.* 348: 781–790. Erratum in: N. Engl. J. Med. 2003; 348: 1508.

Hachamovitch, R., Berman, D.S., Shaw, L.J. et al. (1998). Incremental prognostic value of myocardial perfusion single photon emission computed tomography for the prediction of cardiac death: differential stratification for risk of cardiac death and myocardial infarction. *Circulation* 97: 535–543. Erratum in: Circulation 1998 Jul 14; 98(2): 190.

Hachamovitch, R., Hayes, S., Friedman, J.D. et al. (2003). Determinants of risk and its temporal variation in patients with normal stress myocardial perfusion scans: what is the warranty period of a normal scan? *J. Am. Coll. Cardiol.* 41: 1329–1340.

Mark, D.B., Hlatky, M.A., Harrell, F.E. Jr. et al. (1987). Exercise treadmill score for predicting prognosis in coronary artery disease. *Ann. Intern. Med.* 106: 793–800.

Mark, D.B., Shaw, L., Harrell, F.E. Jr. et al. (1991). Prognostic value of a treadmill exercise score in outpatients with suspected coronary artery disease. *N. Engl. J. Med.* 325: 849–853.

Marwick, T.H., Case, C., Sawada, S. et al. (2001). Prediction of mortality using dobutamine echocardiography. *J. Am. Coll. Cardiol.* 37: 754–760.

Metz, L.D., Beattie, M., Hom, R. et al. (2007). The prognostic value of normal exercise myocardial perfusion imaging and exercise echocardiography: a meta-analysis. *J. Am. Coll. Cardiol.* 49: 227–237.

Mieres, J.H., Gulati, M., Bairey Merz, N. et al., American Heart Association Cardiac Imaging Committee of the Council on Clinical Cardiology; Cardiovascular Imaging and Intervention Committee of the Council on Cardiovascular Radiology and Intervention (2014). Role of noninvasive testing in the clinical evaluation of women with suspected ischemic heart disease: a consensus statement from the American Heart Association. *Circulation* 130: 350–379. Erratum in: Circulation 2014; 130: e86.

Morris, C.K., Ueshima, K., Kawaguchi, T. et al. (1991). The prognostic value of exercise capacity: a review of the literature. *Am. Heart J.* 122: 1423–1431.

Myers, J., Prakash, M., Froelicher, V. et al. (2002). Exercise capacity and mortality among men referred for exercise testing. *N. Engl. J. Med.* 346: 793–801.

Nishime, E.O., Cole, C.R., Blackstone, E.H. et al. (2000). Heart rate recovery and treadmill exercise score as predictors of mortality in patients referred for exercise ECG. *JAMA* 284: 1392–1398.

Nishimura, R.A., Otto, C.M., Bonow, R.O. et al., American College of Cardiology/American Heart Association Task Force on Practice Guidelines (2014). 2014 AHA/ACC guideline for the management of patients with valvular heart disease: a report of the American College of Cardiology/American Heart Association Task Force on Practice Guidelines. *J. Am. Coll. Cardiol.* 63: e57–e185.

Shaw, L.J., Peterson, E.D., Shaw, L.K. et al. (1998). Use of a prognostic treadmill score in identifying diagnostic coronary disease subgroups. *Circulation* 98: 1622–1630.

Shaw, L.J., Mieres, J.H., Hendel, R.H. et al., WOMEN Trial Investigators (2011). Comparative effectiveness of exercise electrocardiography with or without myocardial perfusion single photon emission computed tomography in women with suspected coronary artery disease: results from the What Is the Optimal Method for Ischemia Evaluation in Women (WOMEN) trial. *Circulation* 124: 1239–1249.

Sydó, N., Sydó, T., Gonzalez Carta, K.A. et al. (2018). Prognostic performance of heart rate recovery on an exercise test in a primary prevention population. *J. Am. Heart Assoc.* 7: e008143. https://doi.org/10.1161/JAHA.117.008143.

Weiner, D.A., Ryan, T.J., McCabe, C.H. et al. (1984). Prognostic importance of a clinical profile and exercise test in medically treated patients with coronary artery disease. *J. Am. Coll. Cardiol.* 3: 772–779.

18   Value of Exercise (Stress) ECG Testing Before Engaging in Exercise Programs or Competitive Sports

Bryon A. Gentile and Dennis A. Tighe

Introduction

In general, screening for ischemic heart disease in asymptomatic individuals without known cardiovascular, renal, or metabolic disease with an exercise ECG stress test is not recommended, although it may prove valuable in selected instances. Considerable debate exists as to whether exercise ECG stress testing is helpful in specific populations of asymptomatic adult subjects before beginning vigorous exercise and even more so in young patients prior to beginning competitive sports. This chapter will review the utility of the exercise ECG test in such populations.

Pocket Guide to Stress Testing, Second Edition. Edited by Dennis A. Tighe and Bryon A. Gentile.
© 2020 John Wiley & Sons Ltd. Published 2020 by John Wiley & Sons Ltd.

Proper Interpretation

The exercise ECG stress test has been reported to have a sensitivity and specificity of 68 and 77%, respectively. The number of "false-positive" tests has been a major criticism of this modality in the literature, particularly when applied in low-risk populations. As a result, the value of exercise ECG stress testing prior to engaging in an exercise program or competitive sports has been called into question.

As with any testing modality, the sensitivity and specificity of the test relies upon proper interpretation as well as the population being studied. Chapter 14 provides a thorough review of exercise ECG interpretation, while Chapter 15 covers factors that may cause false-positive and false-negative tests.

Asymptomatic Patients

Current American Heart Association (AHA) and American College of Sports Medicine (ACSM) recommendations do not endorse screening with an exercise ECG test for the presence of occult coronary artery disease (CAD) in asymptomatic individuals at otherwise low-risk of cardiac event as it is known that exercise-related adverse cardiovascular events are often preceded by signs or symptoms. Regular aerobic exercise lessens cardiovascular risk as subjects become increasingly active. Furthermore, the absolute risk of suffering a cardiovascular event (sudden death or acute myocardial infarction [MI]) in an asymptomatic individual during vigorous-intensity exercise is extremely low. The process of exercise pre-participation screening, based on current activity level, screen for signs and symptoms of disease, and desired intensity of exercise, should be at an appropriate but not excessive level, so as not to impose unneeded barriers to performing regular exercise.

- For asymptomatic patients without signs of cardiovascular, renal, or metabolic disease who participate in regular aerobic exercise, medical clearance to continue moderate- or vigorous-intensity exercise is not necessary, and the participant may gradually progress.
- For the asymptomatic patient without signs of cardiovascular, renal, or metabolic disease who does not participate in regular aerobic exercise, medical clearance to initiate light to moderate-intensity exercise is not required; the participant may gradually progress to a vigorous-intensity exercise program.
- For asymptomatic individuals with known disease who already are exercise participants, medical clearance before beginning vigorous-intensity exercise is recommended.
- For asymptomatic patients with known disease, but who do not participate in regular exercise, medical clearance is recommended before beginning an exercise-program of any level of intensity.

Published guidelines and recommendations for screening and exercise ECG testing before exercise participation are available.

Although exercise ECG stress testing prior to beginning or intensifying an exercise program based solely on the presence of risk factors for atherosclerotic cardiovascular disease (ASCVD) *is not recommended currently*, the exercise ECG stress test may have some predictive value in asymptomatic patients with risk factors for CAD.

- The Seattle Heart Watch study found that men with ≥1 risk factor (family history, smoking, hypertension [BP >140/90 mmHg], hypercholesterolemia [total cholesterol >240 mg/dl]) and two abnormalities on exercise ECG stress testing (chest pain, exercise duration <6 minutes, ST-segment depression >1.0 mm, or <90% age-predicated maximal Heart rate [HR]) had a 30-fold increase in 5-year cardiac risk. Exercise testing did not provide predictive value in patients without risk factors.

Thus, exercise testing in asymptomatic men with ≥1 risk factor for CAD may provide further prognostic information to guide risk factor modification, especially for those who do not perform habitual exercise and wish to begin a vigorous-intensity exercise program. It has been postulated that the benefits may extend to women. However, prospective evaluation of outcomes are needed.

Prior to Vigorous Exercise or Competitive Sports

Routine screening of asymptomatic, low-risk individuals with exercise ECG testing is not recommended. For such patients, testing should not be a barrier to beginning an exercise program as the risk of exercise-related morbidity and mortality is very low (see Chapter 19).

The 2010 ACCF/AHA Guideline for Assessment of Cardiovascular Risk in Asymptomatic Adults states that the exercise ECG test may be considered for cardiovascular risk assessment in intermediate-risk asymptomatic adults (including sedentary adults) considering starting a vigorous exercise program (defined as exercise requiring an oxygen uptake ≥ 6 Metabolic equivalents [METs] or 21 ml/kg/min, $\geq 60\%$ Heart rate reserve [HRR] or VO_2R, ≥ 14 Rate of perceived exertion [RPE]), particularly when attention is paid to non-ECG markers such as exercise capacity (Class IIb; level of evidence: B).

The Unites States Preventive Services Task Force concluded that insufficient evidence exists to recommend the use of exercise ECG testing as a screening tool in asymptomatic patents at intermediate to high-risk for ASCVD events.

Exercise ECG testing (as part of an overall medical clearance) may be recommended in individuals with chest pain or dyspnea on exertion to evaluate the risks of exercise or sports participation, as well as, to develop exercise limits and an exercise prescription.

In the United States, routine pre-participation screening of competitive athletes generally consists of obtaining a history and focused physical examination; routine use of the resting 12-lead EGG, much less an exercise ECG test, is not recommended.

Vigorous exertion (including occupational exposures) or competitive sports are not recommended:

- When the expected workload (expressed as METs) exceeds the individual's physical capacity as determined by the exercise ECG test or cardiopulmonary exercise test (CPX).
- When serious ventricular arrhythmias are provoked by exercise, particularly at low workloads.
- Among patients who develop tachyarrhythmias and/or exertional symptoms that are reproducible, until a full medical evaluation has been completed.

Summary
<ul><li>Routine screening for occult CAD with an exercise ECG stress test is not recommended in asymptomatic individuals at low risk of cardiac events.</li><li>Exercise testing prior to a vigorous-intensity exercise program in asymptomatic men with ≥1 risk factor for CAD may provide prognostic information to guide risk factor modification.</li><li>The ACSM's Recommendations for Exercise Pre-participation Health Screening document does not advocate for the routine screening of asymptomatic individuals without known cardiovascular, renal, or metabolic disease prior to a beginning an exercise program. For those individuals already participating in exercise, moderate- or vigorous-intensity activity may be undertaken. For subjects not already participating in regular aerobic exercise, medical clearance is not required to initiate light-to-moderate-intensity physical activity.</li><li>Exercise ECG testing should not be a barrier to exercise in patients with low-risk of exercise-related morbidity and mortality.</li><li>For asymptomatic sedentary patients with known disease, medical clearance is required before beginning an exercise program. For those already participating in an exercise program, medical clearance is recommended before engaging in vigorous-intensity exercise.</li><li>Exercise ECG testing, as part of a medical evaluation, is recommended for symptomatic individuals to prior to initiating any exercise program to evaluate the risks of exercise or sports-related activity, as well as, to develop exercise limits and an exercise prescription.</li></ul>

References

Bruce, R.A., DeRouen, T.A., and Hossack, K.F. (1980). Value of maximal exercise tests in risk assessment of primary coronary heart disease events in healthy men. Five years' experience of the Seattle Heart Watch Study. *Am. J. Cardiol.* 46: 371–378.

Fletcher, G.F., Ades, P.A., Kligfield, P. et al., on behalf of the American Heart Association Exercise, Cardiac Rehabilitation, and Prevention Committee of the Council on Clinical Cardiology, Council on Nutrition, Physical Activity and Metabolism, Council on Cardiovascular and Stroke Nursing, and Council on Epidemiology and Prevention (2013). Exercise standards for testing and training: a scientific statement from the American Heart Association. *Circulation* 128: 873–934.

Gibbons, R.J., Balady, G.J., Bricker, J.T. et al. (2002). ACC/AHA 2002 guideline update for exercise testing: summary article: a report of the American College of Cardiology/American Heart Association Task Force on Practice Guidelines (Committee to Update the 1997 Exercise Testing Guidelines). *Circulation* 106: 1883–1892.

Greenland, P., Alpert, J.S., Beller, G.A. et al. (2010). American College of Cardiology Foundation; American Heart Association. 2010 ACCF/AHA guideline for assessment of cardiovascular risk in asymptomatic adults: a report of the American College of Cardiology Foundation/American Heart Association Task Force on Practice Guidelines. *J. Am. Coll. Cardiol.* 56: e50–e103.

Maron, B.J., Levine, B.D., Washington, R.L. et al. (2015). Eligibility and disqualification recommendations for competitive athletes with cardiovascular abnormalities: task force 2: preparticipation screening for cardiovascular disease in competitive athletes: a scientific statement from the American Heart Association and American College of Cardiology. *J. Am. Coll. Cardiol.* 66: 2356–2361.

Mittleman, M.A., Maclure, M., Tofler, G.H. et al. (1993). Triggering of acute myocardial infarction by heavy physical exertion. Protection against triggering by regular exertion. Determinants of Myocardial Infarction Onset Study Investigators. *N. Engl. J. Med.* 329: 1677–1683.

Mora, S., Redberg, R.F., Cui, Y. et al. (2003). Ability of exercise testing to predict cardiovascular and all-cause death in asymptomatic women: a 20-year follow-up of the lipid research clinics prevalence study. *JAMA* 290: 1600–1607.

Moyer, V.A., Preventive Services, U.S., and Force, T. (2012). Screening for coronary heart disease with electrocardiography: U.S. Preventive Services Task Force recommendation statement. *Ann. Intern. Med.* 157: 512–518.

Riebe, D., Franklin, B.A., Thompson, P.D. et al. (2015). Updating ACSM's recommendations for exercise preparticipation health screening. *Med. Sci. Sports Exerc.* 47: 2473–2479.

Thompson, P.D., Franklin, B.A., Balady, G.J. et al. (2007). Exercise and acute cardiovascular events: placing the risks into perspective: a scientific statement from the American Heart Association Council on Nutrition, Physical Activity, and Metabolism and the Council on Clinical Cardiology. *Circulation* 115: 2358–2368.

19 Exercise Prescriptions for Healthy Individuals and Cardiac Patients

Dennis A. Tighe and Samuel A. E. Headley

Introduction

Aerobic exercise has important health benefits for normal subjects as well as for those with cardiovascular disease. Among patients leading an inactive lifestyle, the incidences of obesity, hyperlipidemia, hypertension, and diabetes are higher than among those more physically active. Abundant data implicates a lack of regular physical activity as a major risk factor for the development of CAD and increased future mortality. With calls for an increasingly active American lifestyle and recognition that regular aerobic exercise confers considerable health benefits, it is important that healthcare professionals understand the planning and implementation of the aerobic exercise prescription for various patient groups. This chapter briefly reviews exercise physiology as it applies to aerobic exercise training, and the principles of exercise prescription for healthy subjects and those with cardiovascular disease.

Pocket Guide to Stress Testing, Second Edition. Edited by Dennis A. Tighe and Bryon A. Gentile.

Physiology of Exercise

The physiology of exercise involves a complex interaction between factors governing control and function of metabolism, muscular contraction, respiration, and the circulatory system.

Metabolism

The energy required for muscular activity is provided from the interaction of three metabolic pathways:

1) *Stored high energy phosphates* (ATP, creatine phosphate): provide energy for high-intensity, short-duration exercise. This energy source is limited by a small storage capacity.
2) *Anaerobic glycolysis* (degradation of glucose to pyruvate or lactate): used to produce energy prior to maximal use of the pathways of oxidative metabolism and when aerobic metabolism cannot provide all the energy needed for exercise. Similar to those of the high-energy phosphates, the maximal capabilities of anaerobic metabolism for exercise capacity are limited. Carbohydrate is the only substrate that can be used as fuel for this pathway.
3) *Oxidative (aerobic) metabolism* produces the vast majority of energy required for exercise through a series of complex metabolic pathways. This pathway can use carbohydrates, fats, or proteins as substrates for energy. Critical to oxidative metabolism is the ability of the cardiopulmonary system to adequately deliver oxygen to contracting skeletal muscle.

Muscle Physiology

Motor units of three types are found in human skeletal muscle.

1) *Type I motor units:* characterized by slow contraction and high capacity for oxidative metabolism. These motor units perform activities requiring prolonged muscle contraction and are well suited for endurance-type activities.
2) *Type IIa motor units:* characterized by fast contraction time and moderate capacity for oxidative metabolism.
3) *Type IIx motor units:* characterized by fast contraction time and low oxidative capacity.
   - Type II motor units are better suited for activities requiring high intensity and short contraction duration (strength and power) in which significant anaerobic metabolism and lactate production occurs.
   - Progressive exercise is characterized by early involvement of Type I units and subsequent recruitment of Type II units. Muscle fatigue occurs due to a complex interplay that occurs between peripheral factors (reduced ATP and increased levels of ADP, inorganic phosphate, and H+) as well as central mechanisms (reduced descending motor drive).

Muscular Contraction

Three types of muscular contractions are recognized:

1) *Isometric (static):* Isometric exercise, characterized by muscular contraction against a fixed resistance and no joint movement, places a greater pressure load than a volume load upon the heart. The cardiac output response to isometric contraction is less than isotonic exercise due to increased resistance. The cardiovascular response to isometric-type work is an increase in both systolic blood pressure (SBP) and diastolic blood pressure (DBP).
2) *Isotonic (dynamic):* Isotonic exercise is characterized by muscular contraction which results in joint movement; it places a volume load on the heart. This action is normally associated with an increase in SBP and either a decrease or no change in DBP.
3) *Resistance (combination of static and dynamic):* Resistance exercise (such as weightlifting) combines features of isometric and isotonic exercise.

Myocardial Oxygen Uptake (VO_{2max})

- Maximal oxygen uptake (in $mlO_2/kg/min$) is the maximum amount of oxygen that a person can use during maximum dynamic exercise while breathing room air at sea level. Physiologically, it represents the amount of oxygen transported and used for cellular metabolism. The term peak oxygen uptake (VO_{2peak}) is used when the criteria for achieving a true maximal test have not been achieved. In most cases deconditioned individuals or individuals with disease do not truly achieve the criteria for a VO_{2max} test during incremental exercise and therefore what they achieve is technically their VO_{2peak}

$$VO_{2max} = \text{Maximum cardiac output} \times \text{Maximum arteriovenous oxygen difference.}$$

- VO_{2max} is related to heart rate (HR) and stroke volume (SV), because

$$\text{Cardiac output}(Q) = SV \times HR$$

- Under normal conditions during dynamic exercise, SV increases until a plateau level is reached, usually at 50–60% of VO_{2max}; HR progressively increases (maximum $HR \approx 220\text{-age} \pm 12\,bpm$), and peripheral oxygen extraction in working muscle beds is increased.
- VO_{2max} is related to a number of factors including amount of muscle mass being exercised, gender (mean values among women are 10–20% less than men), environmental conditions, cardiovascular fitness, and age.
- VO_{2max} is maximum between ages 15 and 30 years. Thereafter, an approximate 9%/decade reduction is found in patients leading a sedentary lifestyle, versus a $\leq 5\%$/decade reduction among the physically active.
- Determination of VO_{2max} for a given individual requires analysis of expired pulmonary gases. This is impractical in most clinical situations (exception cardiopulmonary exercise test [CPX] testing); therefore estimates of VO_{2max} have been derived from peak exercise time during treadmill testing or peak power output achieved with ergometry.

Table 19.1 Normal values for maximal oxygen consumption according to age and gender.[a]

Age (year)	Men (mlO$_2$/kg/min)	Women (mlO$_2$/kg/min)
20–29	47.6 ± 11.3	37.6 ± 10.2
30–39	43.0 ± 9.9	30.9 ± 8.0
40–49	38.8 ± 9.6	27.9 ± 7.7
50–59	33.8 ± 9.1	24.2 ± 6.1
60–69	29.4 ± 7.9	20.7 ± 5.0
70–79	25.8 ± 7.1	18.3 ± 3.6

Source: Adapted with permission from Kaminsky (2015).
[a] Derived from cardiopulmonary exercise testing.

- MET (metabolic equivalent) is the conventional term used to express metabolic energy expenditure (VO$_2$). One MET (3.5 mlO$_2$/kg/min) is the amount of energy expended sitting at rest.
- For clinical exercise testing, METs are estimated from peak exercise workload based upon VO$_2$ data of known populations correlated with exercise intensity and method of exercise.
- Table 19.1 lists normal values for maximal oxygen uptake stratified according to age and gender.

Determinants of Myocardial Oxygen Consumption

- Three determinants of myocardial oxygen consumption are recognized:
  1) Myocardial wall tension (Pressure × Radius/Wall thickness)
  2) Contractility
  3) HR

- Myocardial oxygen consumption is clinically estimated by the product of HR and SBP (rate-pressure product or double product).
  - A linear relationship exists between myocardial oxygen consumption and coronary blood flow.
  - During exercise, coronary blood flow typically increases up to four to sixfold over basal values.
  - Since the normal resting myocardial arteriovenous-O_2 difference is high and relatively fixed, myocardial oxygen delivery must increase in order to meet metabolic demands. Oxygen delivery, therefore, is dependent upon HR, aortic diastolic driving pressure gradient, and coronary vascular resistance. During progressive exercise, vascular resistance in the coronary, cerebrovascular, and exercising muscle declines while vasoconstriction occurs in other vascular beds.

Physiologic Responses to Dynamic Exercise

- In order to perform maximal dynamic exercise, a complex interaction of physiologic events must occur in order to achieve adequate oxygen delivery and uptake.

Pulmonary Response

- Oxygenation of blood is dependent upon adequate alveolar ventilation, efficient gas exchange at the pulmonary capillary-alveolar interface, and the oxygen carrying capacity of the blood.
- At VO_{2max}, alveolar ventilation typically increases 20–25 times over that at rest. With moderate levels of exercise, increased tidal volume is observed. During maximal exertion, increased respiratory rate is required to provide sufficient alveolar ventilation.
- During maximal exercise, respiratory gas exchange is enhanced due to a number of processes. With exercise, the alveolar-pulmonary capillary gradient becomes more favorable for oxygen exchange because the partial pressure of alveolar oxygen is increased and the mixed venous blood O_2 content is reduced due to greater O_2 extraction by

working skeletal muscle. In addition, with exercise, increased recruitment of ventilatory units occurs, resulting in enhanced matching of ventilation and perfusion.

Cardiac Response
Heart Rate

- Among healthy subjects undergoing graded exercise, HR increases in a linear fashion as a function of increasing VO_2 and reaches a plateau just prior to VO_{2max}. The initial rise in HR with exercise is secondary to decreased vagal outflow and is later followed by increased sympathetic nervous system activity.
- Maximum HR response is related to age and is predicted by the formula:

$$\text{Predicted maximum HR} \approx 220 - \text{age}\left(\text{in years}\right) \pm 12\,\text{bpm}.$$

Blood Pressure Response

- SBP rises in a linear fashion with progressive increase in exercise workload due primarily to increasing cardiac output (Q) (peripheral vascular resistance declines with progressive exercise).
- Failure of the SBP to increase ≥ 20–$30\,\text{mmHg}$ with progressive exercise implies inadequate exercise Q, which can result from processes such as left ventricular (LV) outflow tract obstruction, severe myocardial ischemia, or impaired ventricular function of any etiology.
- DBP remains unchanged or may decline slightly in response to dynamic exercise.

Stroke Volume

- With progressive exercise, SV is enhanced by increased venous return and increased myocardial contractility.

- During upright exercise, SV plateaus at 50–60% of VO_{2max} because of the reduction in diastolic filling at higher HRs that is counterbalanced by increased contractility and LVEF.

Cardiac Output

- Q increases in a linear fashion during progressive exercise as a result of increased SV and HR.
- Peak exercise Q is achieved just prior to development of VO_{2max}.

Redistribution of Blood Flow

- At rest, approximately 15–20% of the cardiac output perfuses skeletal muscle beds while the remainder is distributed among other vital organs and the viscera.
- During exercise, vital organ perfusion is maintained. Blood flow to the viscera is dramatically diminished while that to working skeletal muscle is substantially increased and its ability to extract oxygen also increases by approximately threefold.

Exercise Prescription for Healthy Subjects

- The aerobic exercise prescription is an individualized regimen of recommended physical activity and is regulated by the FITT-VP acronym:
  - Frequency
  - Intensity (level of effort)
  - Time (duration of session)
  - Type (mode)
  - Volume and Progression

- The goals of an exercise program depend upon the individual's characteristics and needs. In most cases, an exercise program is structured to accomplish improved physical fitness, enhanced cardiovascular performance, and reduced risk of future cardiovascular disease events.
- The current physical activity guidelines for Americans (PAG) suggest that adults achieve 150–300 minutes per week of moderate-intensity or 75–150 minutes per week of vigorous-intensity aerobic activity. In addition, it is recommended that adults perform muscle-strengthening activities (resistance training and weight-lifting) on two or more days a week. Older adults (age ≥ 65 years) should perform multicomponent physical activity that includes balance training as well as the aerobic and muscle-strengthening activities. Additional health benefits can be realized by performing more activity than is recommended by the PAG.

Risk Stratification Prior to Exercise Program Implementation

- Prior to participation in a structured exercise program, care must be taken to properly evaluate each subject for risk factors and signs of disease that may result in morbidity and mortality from the exercise program while not being overly prohibitive about prescribing exercise among the majority of patients at lower risk, as lack of physical activity is detrimental to overall health. It is well known that the *relative risk* of serious complications from exercise is significantly higher among individuals with known heart disease and during acute vigorous exertion; the *absolute risk* of such events is low and these events are usually preceded by warning signs or symptoms. The current recommendations from the American College of Sports Medicine (ACSM) recognize that scant evidence supports the role of screening examinations or use of diagnostic testing for the purpose of reducing the risk of exercise-related cardiovascular events. Thus, screening should be directed to the highest risk subjects while others at somewhat lower risk may require "medical clearance" from their healthcare provider prior to initiating an exercise program.
- Screening evaluation prior to initiating an exercise program is based on four major categories for assessment:

1) Current level of physical activity
2) Presence of known cardiac, metabolic, or renal disease or existence of signs or symptoms suggestive of disease
3) Desired intensity of the proposed activity
4) Potential hazards due to unaccustomed, high-intensity physical activity

Previous ACSM guidelines recommended that patients be classified as low, moderate, or high risk for atherosclerotic cardiovascular disease (ASCVD) based upon the number of ASCVD risk factors and the presence of signs or symptoms and/or known cardiac, metabolic, pulmonary, or renal disease. The current ACSM recommendations for exercise participation health screening remove the requirement for ASCVD risk factor assessment and focus on directing individuals to seek approval ("medical clearance") to engage in an exercise program from their healthcare professional if signs or symptoms of possible ASCVD exist and/or known cardiovascular (cardiac, peripheral vascular, or cerebrovascular disease), metabolic (type 1 or type 2 diabetes mellitus), or renal disease are present. Of note, it is recommended that subjects with pulmonary disease no longer require automatic referral for medical evaluation because the risks of cardiovascular complications due to exercise are not increased among such patients.

- An algorithm outlining the suggested approach to exercise pre-participation screening is presented in Figure 19.1. These recommendations can be summarized as follows:
  - Physically-active, asymptomatic subjects (with or without known cardiovascular, metabolic, or renal disease): No medical clearance is required for moderate-intensity exercise. Progression to vigorous-intensity activity should be gradual per ASCM guidelines for those without known disease. Patients with known cardiovascular, metabolic, or renal disease should have medical clearance for vigorous-intensity activity.
  - Physically-inactive, asymptomatic subjects without known cardiovascular, metabolic, or renal disease: Medical clearance for light to moderate-intensity exercise is not required; progression to vigorous-intensity activity should be gradual per ASCM guidelines.

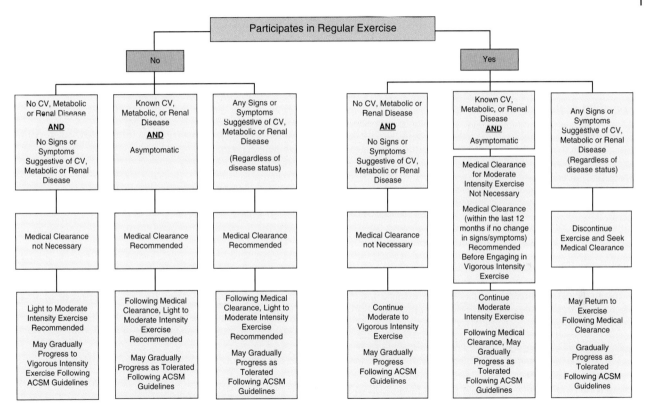

Figure 19.1 Exercise prescription health screening algorithm. *Source:* adapted with permission from Riebe et al. (2015).

- Physically-inactive, asymptomatic patients with known cardiovascular, metabolic, or renal disease: Medical clearance is recommended prior to initiating an exercise program of any intensity.
- Individuals who develop signs or symptoms suggestive of ASCVD with exercise should discontinue exercise and seek medical evaluation.

Principles of the Exercise Prescription

The goal of an exercise program is to enhance cardiovascular wellness and physical fitness. The following recommendations describe essential components of the aerobic exercise prescription.

Frequency of Exercise

For most individuals, exercise should be performed three to seven days per week. If only moderate-intensity exercise is performed, the recommended frequency is five to seven day per week; while three to five days per week is recommended for vigorous-intensity exercise. Some participants may require more or less frequent sessions depending upon exercise intensity and functional capacity.

Intensity of Exercise

- Intensity of aerobic exercise is measured as a percentage of maximal functional capacity, or as a percent of VO_2 reserve (VO_2R). Exercise intensity should be individualized and prescribed at an intensity within the range of 40–89% VO_2R depending upon the level of the subject's fitness. For deconditioned individuals, it may be more appropriate to begin at intensities as low as 30% of VO_2R.
- The intensity of exercise can be monitored using various criteria such as target HR, perceived exertion, or target workload. Intensity of exercise is often determined as a range, thus calculations used for the various parameters must be carried out separately for the lower and upper boundaries of the desired range.

- Exercise intensity can be classified as:
  - Light: 30–<40% HRR or VO2$_R$; 2–<3 METs; 9–11 rate of perceived exertion (RPE)
  - Moderate: 40–<60% HRR or VO2$_R$; 3–6 METs; 12–13 RPE
  - Vigorous: >60% HRR or VO2$_R$; ≥6 METs; ≥14 RPE

HR as a Guide to Exercise Intensity

HR and exercise intensity are related in a linear fashion. The prescribed target HR ranges only provide rough guidelines to follow. Various methods can be used to calculate an appropriate target HR range based on the intensity of exercise:

- Heart rate reserve (HRR) method: Maximal HR determined from an exercise Electrocardiogram ECG test and resting HR are obtained. HRR is the difference between the maximal and resting HR. Using the desired level and range of intensity (%VO$_2$R), the following equation can be used to establish a target HR:

$$\text{Target HR} = \left(\%VO_2R\right)\left(HR_{max} - HR_{rest}\right) + HR_{rest}$$

The HRR method is considered the most accurate method to establish a target HR.

- Percentage of maximal heart (%HR$_{max}$) method: Maximal HR based on age is multiplied by an intensity fraction (related to range of %VO$_2$ R) by using the following equation:

$$\text{Target HR} = \left(\text{intensity fraction}\right)HR_{max}$$

This calculation is simpler than the %HRR and does not require measurement of the resting HR. However, due to the variations in resting HR in the population, this method is considered less accurate than the %HRR method. This method is considered as inappropriate for patients taking HR-limiting drugs.

Target Workload as a Guide to Exercise Intensity

Various methods can be used to establish a target workload:

- %VO$_2$R method:
  To determine the target VO$_2$R, the following formula is used:

$$\text{Target VO}_2\text{R} = \left[\left(\text{VO}_2\text{ max/ peak} - \text{VO}_2\text{rest}\right) \times \text{intensity fraction}\right] + \text{VO}_2\text{rest}$$

- %VO$_{2max}$ method:
  To obtain a target VO$_2$, VO$_{2\text{ max}}$ is multiplied by an intensity fraction using the following formula:

$$\text{Target VO}_2 = \left(\text{intensity fraction}\right)\text{VO}_{2\text{max}}$$

- MET method:
  The MET level associated with various activities is listed in Table 19.2. A range of 40–85% of functional capacity (maximal METs) is prescribed to attain a training effect. The following formula is used to obtain a target MET level:

$$\text{Target MET} = \left[\left(\text{VO}_2\text{ max/ peak}\right)/3.5\,\text{ml}/\text{kg}/\text{min}\right] \times \text{intensity fraction}$$

Initially, prescribed MET levels should be set at the lower end of %maximal capacity. As the participant adapts to this level of exercise, the prescribed MET level is gradually increased to a level approaching 85% of functional capacity.

Table 19.2 Energy requirements of various activities in metabolic equivalents (METs).

Category	Self-care or Home	Occupational	Recreational	Exercise
Very light <3 METs	Personal grooming and hygiene, desk work, dishes, driving car	Sitting (clerical, assembly), standing (store clerk), driving truck	Archery, billiards, golf (cart), horseshoes, shuffleboard	Walking (2 mph), stationary bike (low resistance), very light calisthenics
Light 3–5 METs	Raking, weeding, washing windows, painting, power lawn mowing	Stocking shelves, light carpentry, auto repair, light welding, wallpapering	Dancing, golf (walking), sailing, doubles tennis, horseback riding	Walking (3–4 mph), bicycling (6–8 mph), light calisthenics
Moderate 5–7 METs	Climbing stairs (slowly), light gardening, carrying objects (30–60 lbs), hand lawn mowing on level	Carpentry, pneumatic tools, shoveling dirt	Singles tennis, downhill skiing, basketball, skating, badminton	Walking (4.5–5 mph), bicycling (9–10 mph), swimming
Heavy 7–9 METs	Sawing wood, heavy shoveling, carrying objects (60–90 lb), climbing stairs (moderate speed)	Digging ditches, pick, and shovel use	Canoeing, mountain climbing, fencing, football	Jogging (5 mph), heavy swimming, rowing, bicycling (12 mph), heavy calisthenics
Very heavy >9 METs	Carrying objects (>90 lb), climbing stairs (quickly), shoveling heavy snow, carrying loads upstairs	Lumberjack, heavy laborer	Handball, squash, vigorous basketball, cross-country skiing	Running (≥6 mph), bicycling (≥13 mph), rope jumping

Source: Adapted from Haskell (1978).

Target Intensity Using Perceived Exertion

Rate of Perceived Exertion (RPE)

- The RPE is highly correlated with physiologic responses during progressive exercise and shows little intra-patient variability.
- The most common scale used in clinical practice is that of Borg (Table 19.3). Using the 15-point scale, a perceived exertion of 12–13 corresponds to 60% of target HR while a RPE of 16 corresponds to 85% of target HR.

The Talk Test

With moderate intensity exertion, the subject is usually too winded to sing but remains able to talk. During vigorous exertion, the individual will experience difficulty with maintaining conversation.

Exercise Time (Duration)

- The duration of aerobic exercise should be between 20 and 60 minutes per session to achieve a training effect; if weight-loss is the goal, a duration of up to 90 minutes may be required to achieve the necessary volume of exercise per week. Most programs typically prescribe 20–30 minutes of exercise exclusive of warm-up and cool-down periods. In some cases, multiple shorter sessions (of at least 10 minutes) at the prescribed intensity may be used to attain the desired duration.
- A warm-up period of 5–10 minutes consisting of low-intensity exercise and stretching before the exercise session and a cool-down period during which static stretching is performed following exercise are recommended.
- The warm-up period is designed to minimize exercise-related injury and adapt muscle and joint function to exercise.

Table 19.3 Rate of perceived exertion (RPE).

Borg 15-point scale	Modified Borg 10-point scale
6	0
7 very, very light	0.5 very, very weak
8	1 very weak
9 very light	2 weak
10	3 moderate
11 fairly light	4 somewhat strong
12	5 strong
13 somewhat hard	6
14	7 very strong
15 hard	8
16	9
17 very hard	10 very, very strong
18	maximum
19 very, very hard	
20	

- The cool-down phase involves a gradual decrease in exercise intensity which helps prevent post-exercise hypotension due to venous pooling and allows a gradual reduction in HR toward a resting level.

Type of Activity (Mode of Exercise)

- Any activity requiring the use of large muscle groups that can be maintained for a prolonged period and is aerobic in nature (such as walking, jogging, cycling, rowing, machine stair climbing, etc.) and generally of low impact is recommended.
- The mode of activity should combine aerobic exercise with properly selected resistance exercises (calisthenics, weights).
- The mode of activity should be carefully selected so that it is both enjoyable for the subject and can be accomplished within the appropriate range for the patient.

Volume and Progression

Volume
Volume is computed as the product of frequency, intensity, and time. The goal of a program is to achieve 500–1000 MET-minutes/week. (MET-minutes is computed by taking the MET value for an activity and multiplying it by the number of minutes spent doing the activity.)

Rate of Progression
The aerobic exercise prescription involves three phases of progression: initiation, improvement, and maintenance stages.

Initiation Stage

- The initial conditioning phase is designed to acclimate the participant to the exercise prescription, judge the physiologic and symptomatic response to exercise so that appropriate adjustments can be made, and reinforce compliance with the program.
- Exercise is usually initiated at intensities based on characteristics of the subject: 30% of VO_2R for very deconditioned individuals, 40% of VO_2R for most beginners, and up to 50% of VO_2R for subjects with higher aerobic capacities. At the beginning of the exercise prescription, the duration of aerobic exercise should be at least 10 minutes (20–30 minutes for most participants) with gradual increase in duration as conditioning improves.
- The initiation stage is designed to last four weeks.

Improvement Stage

- During this stage, exercise intensity is gradually increased to the target level to allow for significant improvements in cardiorespiratory fitness without causing overtraining.
- Exercise frequency, intensity, and duration are gradually, but consistently, increased in this stage depending upon patient conditioning.
- The improvement stage usually continues for a period of four to six months.

Maintenance Stage

- This stage generally begins after the first six months of the exercise program.
- Goals and objectives are reviewed and program activities adjusted in order to maintain fitness and compliance.
- Ongoing health maintenance issues are re-emphasized.

Exercise Prescription for the Cardiac Patient

- The general principles of exercise prescription for healthy subjects also apply to those with cardiac disease.
- Among patients with cardiac disease, the largest population encountered is patients with known CAD (post-MI, chronic stable ischemic heart disease, post-percutaneous coronary intervention, post-bypass surgery). Patients with chronic stable heart failure (HF), intermittent claudication, post-heart valve repair or replacement (surgical or percutaneous), and those post-heart transplant surgery or LV-assist device implantation are also candidates for exercise training.
- Patients with CAD demonstrate reduced functional capacity and exercise tolerance in proportion to the extent of atherosclerosis and impairment of LV function. Similarly, patients with non-ischemic heart disease demonstrate limitations in functional capacity and endurance that parallels their underlying cardiovascular function and level of conditioning.
- Exercise training is documented to improve functional capacity and reduce symptoms among patients with ASCVD.
- The goals of exercise training in the coronary patient include:
  - optimization of functional status within limits of disease
  - rehabilitation to perform activities of daily living and appropriate vocational status
  - education for secondary prevention of recurrent events
- The major risks of exercise, especially at a vigorous level, among patients with cardiac disease are sudden death and other cardiac complications (arrhythmia, HF, chest pain, MI). Therefore, a medical evaluation and assessment of functional status prior to an exercise program are required.

Risk Stratification Prior to Exercise

- Among patients with CAD, the risk of sudden death and other clinical manifestations of CAD is related to the degree of LV functional impairment and residual myocardial ischemia. Other factors include age, presence of ventricular or atrial arrhythmia, valvular heart disease, and other non-cardiac co-morbidities.
- A medical evaluation including clinical history, physical examination, and review of the baseline ECG is required prior to entering an exercise program. Many programs conduct a baseline symptom-limited exercise ECG test prior to beginning the exercise program. This evaluation provides significant information pertaining to baseline functional status and allows initial determination of program intensity.
- Patients with significant resting LV dysfunction, decompensated HF, and/or ischemia at rest are not candidates for exercise training until these processes are addressed and treated.
- Patients with inducible ischemia at a low exercise workload (see Chapter 17) should be referred for more detailed cardiovascular evaluation prior to beginning an exercise program.
- Patients with standard contraindications to exercise testing (see Chapter 4) should defer exercise training until these problems are addressed and resolved.
- Based upon medical evaluation and the baseline exercise ECG stress test, patients can be stratified into risk classifications prior to exercise training (Table 19.4).

Cardiac Rehabilitation

Cardiac rehabilitation is a multi-disciplinary, multi-faceted program that provides a systematic approach to exercise training and risk factor modification that incorporates three phases: Inpatient (phase I); Early outpatient period (phase II); and Late outpatient period (phase III).

Table 19.4 Risk classification for exercise training.

Class A: Apparently healthy individuals

  Generally, no activity restrictions

  Should follow basic American College of Sports Medicine (ACSM) guidelines for initiation and progression (see Figure 19.1)

  Monitored setting not required

Class B: Presence of known, but stable, CV disease with low-risk for complications of vigorous exercise

  Clinically stable patients with CV disease who meet the following criteria:

    New York Heart Association (NYHA) class I or II

    Exercise capacity ≥6 metabolic equivalents (METs)

    No overt heart failure (HF) symptoms

    No evidence of angina pectoris or exercise-induced ischemia

    No significant ventricular ectopy

    Appropriate blood pressure (BP) response to baseline exercise Electrocardiogram (ECG) stress test

  Medical supervision and monitoring of ECG and BP during early phases of exercise training are indicated

Class C: Moderate to high risk for complications during exercise

  Patients with known CV disease with moderate to high risk characteristics:

    New York Heart Association (NYHA) class ≥III

    Exercise capacity <6 METs

    Angina pectoris or exercise-induced ischemia at <6 METs

    Significant ventricular ectopy

    Inappropriate BP response to baseline exercise ECG stress test

    Prior primary cardiac arrest outside of acute myocardial infarction (MI) setting

  Medical supervision and continuous monitoring of heart rate (HR) and BP is required during exercise training until safety is established

Class D: Unstable CV disease

  Patients who require activity restriction

  Exercise training is contraindicated

Inpatient Rehabilitation (Phase I)

- The inpatient phase includes patients with recent MI (within one to two days), those who have had cardiac surgery, and those with HF.
- Phase I typically begins with sitting in a chair twice-a-day to induce gravitational stress and performing passive range of motion exercises and progresses to slow indoor walking (approximately 5–10 minutes, two to four times per day) and independent ambulation as tolerated.
- During this phase, the patient is monitored for altered hemodynamic parameters (BP and HR) and symptomatic status during and after activity.
- In recent years, as inpatient hospital lengths of stay for cardiac patients have dramatically shortened (less deconditioning), this phase has become compressed and often this process is used to screen patients for participation in the outpatient phases of cardiac rehabilitation along with providing information on appropriate post-hospital discharge activity.
- Efforts toward and information to modify risk factors for ASCVD are initiated during this phase.
- The patient is provided with guidelines for home activity, reporting of symptoms, sexual activity, and return to vocation.
- A pre-discharge submaximal exercise ECG test may be obtained to guide further therapy and home activities and plan future phases of cardiac rehabilitation.

Early Outpatient Phase (Phase II)

- Phase II begins typically within two weeks of hospital discharge and continues for approximately 12 weeks (total 36 sessions).
- Ideally, phase II programs should be administered in a hospital setting or in a medical facility with immediate access to ECG monitoring and emergency cardiac care.

- This phase involves crafting of an individual exercise prescription using the FITT-VP recommendations to increase aerobic activity via a progressive increase (1 MET every two weeks) in the distance and pace of walking. Resistance and balance (as required) exercises are also incorporated in this prescription.
- HR and rhythm are obtained before, during, and after exercise. Blood pressure response to exercise and RPE should also be monitored. An exercise session should be terminated when indicated to prevent adverse outcomes (Table 19.5).
- Exercise intensity for patients with stable angina pectoris should be set at 10–15 bpm lower than the ischemic threshold documented with the exercise ECG test.
- The frequency of exercise generally should be three to four sessions per week.
- Exercise duration can vary between 15 and 60 minutes per session depending upon the patient's functional capacity and rate of progression.
- A symptom-limited exercise ECG test is performed at the end of phase II.
- In addition to the exercise prescription, the phase II program includes education to modify the patient's ASCVD risk factors, nutritional counseling, review of medication adherence and compliance, weight management, evaluation of blood lipids, diabetes management, tobacco cessation, and psychosocial assessment and management, with the goals to modify risk and preparation for return to vocational activities.
- Suggested criteria for successful completion of phase II include:
  - Stable medical status:
    1) angina stable or absent
    2) normal hemodynamic response to exercise
    3) normal or unchanged ECG response to exercise
    4) controlled resting HR (<90 bpm) and BP (<130/80 mm Hg).
  - Functional capacity ≥5 METs.
  - Clear understanding of individual limitations, risk factors for ASCVD, compliance with medications, appropriate dietary modifications. and the basic pathophysiology of underlying disease on the part of the patient.
  - Adequate physical fitness.

Table 19.5 Indications for termination of a symptom-limited exercise test.

Absolute

- ST-segment elevation ≥1 mm in leads without pre-existing q-waves (other than leads V1, aVL, or aVR)
- Drop in systolic blood pressure (SBP) ≥10 mmHg with an increase in work load, or if SBP decreases below the value obtained in the same position prior to testing when accompanied by other evidence of ischemia
- Moderate-to-severe angina
- Central nervous system symptoms (ataxia, dizziness, near-syncope)
- Signs of poor perfusion (cyanosis, pallor, confusion)
- Sustained ventricular tachycardia (VT) or other arrhythmia, including second- or third-degree atrioventricular (AV) block, that interferes with normal maintenance of cardiac output with exercise
- Failure of monitoring equipment (electrocardiogram [ECG], blood pressure [BP])
- Subject's desire to stop

Relative

- Marked ST-segment displacement or QRS changes such as excessive ST-segment depressions (>2 mm horizontal or downsloping contour) or marked axis shift in a patient with suspected ischemia
- Drop in SBP ≥10 mmHg (persistently below the value obtained in the same position prior to testing) with an increase in work load in the absence of other evidence of ischemia
- Increasing chest pain
- Fatigue, shortness of breath, wheezing, leg cramps, or claudication
- Arrhythmias other than sustained VT, including multifocal ventricular premature contractions (VPCs), ventricular triplets, SVT, or bradyarrhythmias that have the potential to become more complex or to interfere with hemodynamic stability
- Hypertensive response (SBP >250 mmHg and/or DBP >115 mmHg)
- Development of bundle branch block or intraventricular conduction delay that cannot be distinguished from VT
- SpO_2 ≤ 80%

Adapted with permission from: Clinical exercise testing and interpretation, in *ACSM's Guidelines for Exercise Testing and Prescription* (2018, p. 125).

Late Outpatient Phase (Phase III)

- Phase III, which is an enduring unmonitored exercise program, typically begins 12 or more weeks after hospital discharge.
- Only patients with absent or clinically stable angina, clinically stable arrhythmia, normal hemodynamic response to exercise, functional capacity ≥5 METs, and previous medical evaluation should participate in a Phase III program.
- Phase III programs typically continue for 3–12 months, with the goal of enhancing exercise endurance training and functional capacity beyond 8 METs so that the patient can resume a full lifestyle.
- As compared to Phase II programs, Phase III programs are less structured, need not be offered in a hospital setting, and require less staff supervision.
- Within the first three to six months of participation, exercise intensity is gradually increased to achieve 50–85% of functional capacity during three to four sessions per week.
- Once desired functional capacity (≥8 METs) has been achieved, maintenance of and compliance with this level of exercise is the goal.
- Phase III programs should reinforce necessary lifestyle modifications to reduce risk of future complications of ASCVD.

Patients with Heart Failure with Reduced Ejection Fraction

- HF patients have limited exercise capacity that in most cases is often multifactorial. Factors which can limit exercise capacity among patients with HF include:
  - Degree of LV dysfunction
  - Increased central venous pressure
  - Impaired skeletal muscle perfusion
  - Chronic sympathetic nervous system overactivity

- Reduced skeletal muscle mass (atrophy)
- Co-existing arrhythmias and valvular heart disease
- Deconditioning
- Co-morbid conditions (renal dysfunction and electrolyte abnormalities, anemia, etc.)

Prognosis

- Prognosis in HF is related to functional status. Directly measured $VO_{2max} < 10$ ml/kg/min and VE/V_{CO2} slope ≥ 45 is associated with poor prognosis, while $VO_{2max} > 20$ ml/kg/min and VE/V_{CO2} slope ≤ 29.9 is associated with excellent prognosis.
- Consistently it has been shown that prognosis is not related to the resting LVEF taken in isolation.

Exercise Training

- Medically stable patients with NYHA class II and III HF (exercise capacity >3 METs and without exercise-induced ischemia or arrhythmia) are eligible to participate in exercise training programs. Exercise training in such patients is documented to be safe and well-tolerated.
- The benefits of exercise training among patients with HF include increased functional capacity (VO_{2max}), increased maximum arteriovenous O_2 difference, decreased lactate production, increased LVEF, positive LV remodeling, increased skeletal muscle blood flow and function, increased ventilatory efficiency, reduced HF hospitalizations, and improved quality of life.
- Interestingly, numerous studies have failed to demonstrate significant improvements in central hemodynamic measurements with exercise training.
- The exercise intensity initially should be moderate (50–60% VO_{2max} or %HRR) for brief intervals (two to six minutes) with short rest periods in between. Total exercise time should be 30–40 minutes per session. RPE scale values of 12–14 (on the 15-point scale) are recommended because the HR response may be impaired among HF patients.

- Training intensity and duration can be gradually advanced in accord with hemodynamic response to exercise and symptomatic status. While most training is focused on aerobic exercise, addition of resistance training can provide positive benefits to selected patients.
- Blood pressure and heart rhythm should be closely monitored during exercise because of the risks of exercise and/or medicine-induced hypotension and ventricular arrhythmia.
- Exercise programs for patients with HF can be center-based (most common) or based at home, where "tele-rehabilitation" methods can be used for selected patients.

Summary

- Aerobic exercise has been shown to benefit both healthy subjects and those with cardiovascular disease.
- A lack of regular physical activity is associated with increased incidence of obesity, hyperlipidemia, hypertension, and diabetes.
- Sedentary individuals are at increased risk for the development of CAD and future cardiac mortality.
- As the American lifestyle becomes increasingly active, it is important for healthcare professionals to become involved in the planning and implementation of safe and appropriate exercise programs for their patients.
- The PAG for Americans provides recommendations on the types and amounts of activity associated with improved cardiovascular health and reduced risk of future ASCVD events.
- Exercise physiology involves a complex interaction between factors which govern metabolism, muscular contraction, respiration, and the circulatory system.
- The aerobic exercise prescription is an individualized regimen of physical activity consisting of the FITT-VP scheme.

- The goals of the exercise program include reduction of sedentary behavior, improved physical fitness, enhanced cardiovascular performance, and reduced risk of future cardiovascular disease.
- Prior to participation in an exercise program patients with suspected or proven cardiac, metabolic or renal disease must be carefully evaluated to determine the need for medical clearance prior to starting the program or changing to a vigorous intensity.
- This information allows design of an individualized exercise prescription of appropriate initial intensity and volume.
- A training effect can be achieved with as little as 20–30 minutes of exercise at a frequency of three times per week; greater volume and intensity of exercise is association with added health benefits
- A warm-up period and cool-down phase are important components of the exercise session.
- The progression of the exercise prescription is based upon the patient's functional response to exercise.
- Early phases of cardiac rehabilitation require close monitoring of symptomatic status and hemodynamic response to exercise, especially among patients classified as being at risk levels B and C. Later phases are less structured and require less medical supervision.

References

Carter, S., Hartman, Y., Holder, S. et al. (2017). Sedentary behavior and cardiovascular disease risk: mediating mechanisms. *Exerc. Sport Sci. Rev.* 45: 80–86.

Fletcher, G.F., Ades, P.A., Kligfield, P. et al., American Heart Association Exercise, Cardiac Rehabilitation, and Prevention Committee of the Council on Clinical Cardiology, Council on Nutrition, Physical Activity and Metabolism, Council on Cardiovascular and Stroke Nursing, and Council on Epidemiology and Prevention (2013). Exercise standards for testing and training: a scientific statement from the American Heart Association. *Circulation* 128: 873–934.

Garber, C.E., Blissmer, B., Deschenes, M.R. et al., American College of Sports Medicine. American College of Sports Medicine position stand (2011). Quantity and quality of exercise for developing and maintaining cardiorespiratory, musculoskeletal, and neuromotor fitness in apparently healthy adults: guidance for prescribing exercise. *Med. Sci. Sports Exerc.* 43: 1334–1359.

Haskell, W.L. (1978). Design and implementation of cardiac conditioning programs. In: *Rehabilitation of the Coronary Patient* (eds. N.K. Wenger and H.K. Hellerstein), 214–215. New York: Wiley.

Kaminsky, L.A., Arena, R., and Myers, J. (2015). Reference standards for cardiorespiratory fitness measured with cardiopulmonary exercise testing: data from the fitness registry and the importance of exercise national database. *Mayo Clin. Proc.* 90: 1515–1523.

Physical Activity Guidelines Advisory Committee (2018). *2018 Physical Activity Guidelines Advisory Committee Scientific Report*. Washington, DC: U.S. Department of Health and Human Services.

Reibe, D., Ehrman, J., Liguori, G., and Magal, M. (eds.) (2018). *ACSM's Guidelines for Exercise Testing and Prescription*, 10e. Philadelphia: Wolters Kluwer.

Riebe, D., Franklin, B.A., Thompson, P.D. et al. (2015). Updating ACSM's recommendations for exercise preparticipation health screening. *Med. Sci. Sports Exerc.* 47: 2473–2479. Erratum in: Med. Sci. Sports Exerc. 2016;48: 579.

Ross, R., Blair, S.N., Arena, R. et al., American Heart Association Physical Activity Committee of the Council on Lifestyle and Cardiometabolic Health; Council on Clinical Cardiology; Council on Epidemiology and Prevention; Council on Cardiovascular and Stroke Nursing; Council on Functional Genomics and Translational Biology; Stroke Council (2016). Importance of assessing cardiorespiratory fitness in clinical practice: a case for fitness as a clinical vital sign: a scientific statement from the American Heart Association. *Circulation* 134: e653–e699.

20 Computer Technology in the Field of Exercise ECG Stress Testing

Dennis A. Tighe

Introduction

Modern stress ECG systems incorporate computer technology that automates the actual performance of the stress test based upon operator-defined parameters, controls data input and signal processing, and allows more sophisticated interpretation of stress-derived data beyond that obtained from simple manual examination of the ST-segment response to stress. In addition, clinical and exercise (stress) ECG testing variables can be analyzed by computer programs that allow comparison to known databases for determination of post-test (posterior) probability of coronary artery disease (CAD) and for prognostic implications. This chapter briefly reviews computer technology as it relates to the field of exercise (stress) ECG testing.

Computer-Driven Automated Performance of the Exercise ECG Test

- Current stress ECG systems possess computer systems which automate the performance of the entire exercise and recovery portion of the stress test and archive data according to the specifications of the stress laboratory and the institution.
- Most systems allow efficient keyboard or touchscreen entry of patient data and protocol selection and are designed so that combinations of keystrokes or screen touches perform specific functions during system operation.
- Modern systems also permit integration of data from peripheral devices that can used during the stress testing session such as automated blood pressure (BP) and pulse oximetry systems. Wireless transmission of the data to the stress system, eliminating the need for a tethered cable, is an option on some systems.

Test Preparation Phase

- Variables which can be entered and customized prior to performance of a stress test include:
  - *Procedure:* represents the set of parameters that defines how the stress test will be performed. Parameters include: ECG lead set, alarm settings, various prompts, analog output configuration, and ST slope and level.
  - *Exercise device* (treadmill, ergometer, or pharmacological test).
  - *Testing protocol* (see Chapter 5).
  - *Patient data* (name, age, sex, height, and weight, medications, cardiac risk factors). From this data the system automatically calculates age-predicted maximal heart rate (MHR) and target heart rate (HR) (usually 85% MHR for symptom-limited testing and 70% MHR for post-MI testing).
  - Monitoring health professional.
  - Final report template.

- An electrode check is performed after the electrodes are applied and the patient cable is connected to the stress system (exception: use of wireless communication) to assess adequacy of skin preparation. It is extremely important that skin preparation is adequate since the quality of the final analysis of the stress ECG data is critically dependent upon good signal input, so that noise and artifact is minimized (see Chapter 2).
- After a standard resting 12-lead ECG has been obtained, the above parameters have been selected and properly entered, and adequacy of skin preparation has been verified, the exercise (stress) ECG system is started.

Exercise Phase

- The exercise phase begins in accord with the particular protocol chosen by the operator. The computer system will automatically advance the speed and grade of the treadmill unless manually over-ridden by the operator.
- A continuous display of the current stage number, elapsed time of the current stage, total elapsed time of exercise, current HR, and treadmill speed and grade is shown. Additional parameters such as ST level or slope, rate of perceived exertion, metabolic equivalents (METs) or Watts achieved, BP trend, HR trend, rate-pressure product, and SpO_2 can be configured and displayed throughout the test. Several of these parameters can be presented in graphical format.
- During each stage of exercise, from 3- to 16-lead sets (vendor-dependent) can be monitored continuously and a 12-lead ECG printed out or captured in the system (if paperless interpretation occurs) at pre-defined intervals (usually just prior to a completed exercise stage). These automated systems allow for acquisition of a 12-lead ECG and/or rhythm strip at any time during the monitoring period. In addition, current systems provide an algorithm for detection of ectopic beats and arrhythmias and a "hold screen" function that allows more detailed examination of a particular beat or group of beats.
- All systems allow for manual over-ride of protocols and discontinuation of exercise, holding of a particular stage for a longer period of time, or stage advancement.

Recovery Phase

- Upon completion of exercise, the recovery phase is entered. The treadmill gradually slows down and reduces in grade until it is stopped by the operator. The HR, ECG lead set, and elapsed time of recovery are continuously displayed until discontinued by the operator.
- A final report which contains the variables pre-specified by the operator can be generated by the computer system. Modern systems allow for digital storage of information from the current exercise (stress) ECG test for later review and analysis, retrieval of prior stress ECG tests for comparison, dissemination and sharing of information to various sites via the electronic health record or Picture archiving and communication system (PACS) system, or for research purposes.

Data Processing

- In order to process the large amount of data obtained during an exercise stress ECG test and enhance the reading and measurement of the stress ECG, all systems employ computer algorithms for signal and data processing.
- Although the specifics of a particular algorithm are unique to a given system/vendor, certain processes are common to all available systems:

Signal Acquisition

- Analog ECG signals from the body surface enter the stress system via a patient cable or wireless communication which presents them to a preamplifier for digital conversion (numerical voltage values in binary number format at repeated specific time intervals).

- Most current systems sample the ECG at rate of 500–1000 samples/s (Hz) with an input signal resolution of about 5 µV/LSB.
- The digitized signals from the input electrode signals are converted to a 12-lead set (Standard 12-lead, Cornell 12-lead, or Cabrera 12-lead) pre-determined by the operator based upon the computer algorithm.
- Digitized signals are sent to a series of filters to reduce "noise" (any electrical signal foreign to the ECG or that distorts the waveform).
- Noise may emanate from a variety of sources (Table 20.1).
- The most important means to prevent noise is meticulous skin preparation.
- Important sources of noise, especially at higher exercise workloads, are those produced by skeletal muscle and respiratory variation. Digital filtering techniques are applied to reduce these forms of artifact.

Table 20.1 Sources of noise associated with the Exercise (Stress) ECG.

Source of noise	Nature of noise	Means of correction
Skeletal muscle contraction	High frequency	Signal averaging, Low-pass filtering, Loosen grip on handrails
Respiratory variability	Low-frequency baseline wander	High-pass filtering, Cubic spline curve fitting
Electrical line frequency interference	60 cycle interference	Change electric lines, Remove sources of interference, Protected cables/outlets, 60 Hz notch filter
Poor electrode contact	Baseline drift, Low-frequency	Meticulous skin preparation

Muscle Noise

- Muscle noise artifact is due to activation of skeletal muscle groups and tends to be of high frequency. It is also random in nature and, therefore, not synchronous in all leads.
  Approaches to reduce muscle artifact include:
  - Signal averaging (averaging multiple beats reduces the effect of random, unrelated noise).
  - Low-pass filtering.
  - Time-varying low-pass filtering (slope of the ECG signal is sensed and this slope is used to control the band-width of a low-pass filter).

Respiratory Variation

- Respiration leads to wandering of the ECG baseline that varies with the respiratory cycle. Strategies employed to reduce the effect of baseline wandering include high-pass filtering and cubic spline curve fitting.
- Conventional high-pass filtering seeks to block low-frequency signals which cause baseline wander; however, distortion of the ST-segment may occur if filter response is non-linear.
- Technologic advances in digital signal processing have permitted the development of linear high-pass filtering, which prevents ST-segment distortion.
- Cubic spline curve fitting attempts to approximate (smooth) the ECG baseline by fitting a curve through the isoelectric points of successive waveforms.

Recognition of the ECG Complexes (QRS Detection)

The QRS complex, because of its large amplitude, is the most easily detected portion of the ECG input signal.

- QRS detection may be based on QRS amplitude, frequency, morphology, or rate of voltage change of a specific portion of the QRS complex.
- The ECG is sampled at periodic intervals for a specific time period in order to select a dominant beat.
- Algorithms are employed to exclude abnormally tall T-waves (which would result in double counting) and ectopic beats.

Beat Alignment and Classification

- Once a dominant beat is classified, a fiducial (reference) point is defined in each beat in each ECG lead so that other "normal" beats can be aligned in reference to this point.
- After aligning beats by a specific fiducial point, signal averaging is performed.
- A requirement for the averaging process to be accurate is that individual beats to be averaged must be as similar in morphology as possible to the designated dominant beat.
- Various algorithms are used to define a beat as being "normal." The variables most commonly assessed include QRS duration, R-R interval, R-wave amplitude, and template-matching in relation to the dominant beat.
  - Ventricular ectopic beats and aberrantly conducted beats usually have a prolonged QRS duration in relation to the dominant beat and are excluded based on morphology.
  - Premature beats that possess an ectopic R-R interval that is $\geq 20\%$ less than the mean R-R interval or with dissimilar polarity to the dominant beat are excluded.
  - Beats which show poor correlation coefficient compared to the dominant beat are excluded with template matching.
  - These criteria are updated continuously by the computer system throughout the duration of the stress test in order to determine which (normal) beats are used for averaging and for reporting ectopic rate and frequency.

Signal Averaging

- Following alignment and classification of beats, signal averaging is employed to diminish noise and create average beats for each ECG lead to allow more accurate measurement of ECG parameters.
- Average beats can be constructed using either mean or median values.
- The median value has greater central tendency and is less affected by extreme values as compared to the mean. The level of random noise reduction, however, is lessened when the median value is used.
- Most systems form an average beat from analysis of ECG data for each lead every 10 seconds.

Waveform Recognition and Measurement

- Waveform recognition requires that accurate determination of the beginning and end of all intervals of the cardiac cycle be achieved throughout the stress test.
- Most stress systems identify the beginning and end of the QRS complex on the basis of change in spatial vector velocity in multiple ECG leads.
- Location of the isoelectric point is most important because most ST-segment measurements are made with reference to this baseline.
- The isoelectric point is usually identified as the minimum level of activity occurring just prior to the QRS complex. In some cases an isoelectric point cannot be located due to noise and/or abnormality or delay in atrial repolarization. In this situation, the isoelectric point is assigned a location prior to the detected QRS complex by a certain time interval determined by the computer algorithm.
- Following identification of the isoelectric point, each signal averaged beat is adjusted so that the isoelectric baseline is maintained.

- The J-point is placed at the junction of the end of the QRS activity and the beginning of the ST-segment based upon identifying the first point after the latest peak activity of the QRS spatial velocity vector that drops below a predefined threshold for a specified time period.
- From identification and definition of these points, analysis of ST-segment parameters, such as the ST level and ST slope, can be generated for each ECG lead.

Computerized Analysis of ST-Segment Response to Stress

- With properly obtained and processed signal-averaged data, digital measurements have been shown to equally or more accurate, and significantly more reproducible, than similar measurements manually obtained.
- In spite of the advantages offered by digital signal processing, meticulous skin preparation, appropriate lead placement, and oversight of an experienced physician are required to maximize diagnostic yield.
- Various algorithms and semi-automated computer programs for analysis of ST-segment parameters are available; some have been used in large-scale multicenter clinical trials for quantitative analysis and interpretation of large volumes of stress ECG tests.
- In an effort to improve the diagnostic yield of the exercise ECG compared to manual inspection of the ST-segment response to stress, a number of investigators have proposed various parameters that can be derived from computer analysis of the ST-segment data.

ST Integral (Area)

Sheffield and colleagues computed the time-voltage integral of the ST-segment beginning at the end of the QRS complex and continuing until the isoelectric baseline was reached or 80 ms had elapsed following the QRS. An ST integral more negative than $-7.5\,\mu\text{V-s}$ was considered as abnormal, yielding a test sensitivity of 81% and a specificity of 95% for distinguishing normal control subjects from those with a clinical diagnosis of CAD.

ST Index

McHenry and colleagues measured the amplitude of ST-segment depression at 60–70 ms beyond the R-wave peak and the slope of the ST-segment between 70 and 110 ms. The algebraic sum of the ST-segment depression in mm and the ST slope in mV/s (defined as the ST index) was considered abnormal if a value less than zero ("negative index") was obtained. The reported sensitivity for detection of angiographic CAD was 82% (lower in patients with isolated right coronary artery or left circumflex disease) and specificity was 95%.

ST-60 Amplitude

Simoons and Hugenholtz found that the amplitude of ST-segment depression measured at 60 ms after the QRS complex adjusted for HR (ST-60) improved the sensitivity of the exercise ECG test compared to standard visual interpretation. These investigators reported a sensitivity of 70–81% (training and test groups respectively) and specificity of 93% for separation of normal subjects from those with angiographic CAD.

Hollenberg Treadmill Score

Hollenberg and colleagues measured the area under the curves of J-point deviation and ST-segment slope in leads aVF and V_5 and summed them. This sum was then divided by the product of exercise duration (in minutes) and percentage age-predicted maximal heart rate (APMHR) achieved to yield a "treadmill score" in a group of patients with chest pain and known coronary anatomy.

$$\text{Treadmill Score} = \frac{\text{Area of J-point} + \text{ST-slope curves}}{\text{Exercise duration} \times \% \text{APMHR}}$$

A score < -4 was defined as a "positive test." In general, patients with more severe angiographic CAD had more negative treadmill scores.

Heart Rate-Adjusted Indexes of ST-Segment Depression

ST/HR Slope

- Linear regression analysis of the maximal (peak) rate-related change in ST-segment depression (ST/HR slope) among all monitored leads has been shown to accurately identify patients with 0-, 1-, 2-, or 3-vessel CAD when bicycle ergometry (characterized by a gradual HR increment with each successive stage) is employed as the method of stress.
- When the standard Bruce treadmill exercise protocol is performed, HR increments between stages are large and the observed accuracy of the ST/HR slope is diminished.
- Okin and Kligfield and colleagues have identified the limitation of this method when using the standard Bruce protocol and developed a modification of the Bruce protocol (the Cornell protocol) that produces a smaller HR increment between stages while maintaining similar overall workload. These investigators have shown that this modified protocol allows calculation of statistically valid, highly reproducible ST/HR slopes in almost all patients.
- A maximum ST/HR slope measured 60 ms after the J-point of 2.4 μV/beat/min is reported to be a significantly more sensitive partition than visual analysis of the ST-segment in discriminating normal subjects from those with CAD. Furthermore, an ST/HR slope >6 μV/beat/min is reported to be a sensitive and specific indicator of triple vessel or functionally significant double vessel CAD.

ΔST/HR Index

- The ΔST/HR index represents the *average* change of the ST-segment depression measured at 60 ms after the J-point with HR throughout exercise rather than the *peak* rate of ST-segment change with HR at the highest exercise workload (ST/HR slope).
- Kligfield and colleagues studied well-defined patient groups with low pretest likelihood of CAD to determine ΔST/HR partitions defining the upper 95% of normal. Patients with high likelihood of disease and those with angiographically-proved CAD were then studied to determine the sensitivity of this method to detect CAD.
- These investigators reported that a positive index (defined as a value ≥1.6 µV/beat/min) exhibited high sensitivity among patients with high likelihood of CAD while maintaining high specificity among patients with low likelihood of CAD.
- Specificity of this index (and the ST/HR slope) is lower among heterogeneous populations such as those with a high prevalence of non-ischemic cardiac diseases that may affect repolarization, such as with valvular heart disease or cardiomyopathy, and among those with chest pain and angiographically-normal coronary arteries.

Rate-Recovery Loop

- The rate-recovery loop represents a construct of the recovery phase pattern of absolute ST-segment depression plotted with reference to changing HR.
- A normal rate-recovery loop is characterized by a clockwise loop of ST-segment depression as a function of HR during exercise and recovery.
- An abnormal rate-recovery loop is characterized by a counterclockwise loop of ST-segment depression as a function of HR during exercise and recovery.
- This index has been reported to improve the detection of CAD as compared to the standard exercise ECG test and to be an independent predictor of future cardiac events among asymptomatic subjects.

- The combination of an abnormal rate-recovery loop and a positive ΔST/HR index is reported to identify a small group of asymptomatic patients at increased risk (RR = 6.0) of future coronary events within four-years.

ST/HR Hysteresis

- ST segment depression/HR hysteresis is a method to integrate exercise and recovery phase ST/HR analysis by determining the prevailing direction and average magnitude of the hysteresis in ST-segment depression against HR during the first consecutive three minutes of recovery after exercise.
- Lehtinen and colleagues and others have shown that ST/HR hysteresis may provide higher diagnostic and prognostic test accuracy in comparison to that found for standard visual ST-segment depression criteria and for the ST/HR index. This method may provide increased discriminative power in women.

Although these HR-adjusted indexes have been shown to increase the sensitivity to detect CAD (primarily by reclassifying equivocal ECG responses) while preserving test specificity as compared to standard visual ST-segment criteria, some investigators have found varying results. In fact, some investigators have reported that HR-adjusted ST-segment indexes did not provide additional diagnostic information beyond that available from standard visual analysis of the ST-segment using the Bruce protocol. In general, these methods have not been widely adopted for clinical use due to lack of familiarity among clinicians and because further prospective evaluation is required.

Other Approaches to Identify Exercise-Induced Ischemia

- Computerized analysis of stress ECG data other than the ST-segment response to exercise to improve the diagnostic power of the exercise ECG test for identifying myocardial ischemia has been proposed.

- Investigators have studied parameters such as QRS slopes and high-frequency QRS analysis of depolarization abnormalities; they report equivalent or improved diagnostic accuracy for detection of exercise-induced ischemia compared to conventional ST-segment analysis.
- Similar to computerized analysis of the ST-segment, these methods have not been adopted for clinical use as further prospective evaluation is required.

Computer Applications to Estimate Post-Test Probability of CAD

- Computer-based programs which employ multivariate methods to estimate the post-test probability of CAD following exercise testing have been studied.
- CADENZA (computer assisted diagnosis and evaluation of CAD) uses Bayesian analysis and employs a database of >60 000 patients to analyze and report the results of various clinical factors (age, sex, character of chest pain, and traditional cardiac risk factors) and non-invasive test results relative to the diagnosis of CAD. A high correlation between CADENZA estimated post-test likelihood of disease and angiographically-proved CAD has been demonstrated.
- Logistic regression-derived algorithms, unlike those based on Bayes' theorem, do not assume that individual observations analyzed are all stochastically independent. These algorithms have been developed because methods that assume independence may produce larger errors when a greater number of variables are used to estimate probability.
- Although variable clinical results have been observed, certain investigators report that logistic regression analysis-derived algorithms are modestly more accurate in predicting post-test likelihood of CAD than are approaches such as CADENZA.
- These computer-based algorithms appear to enhance the diagnostic information available from the exercise ECG test; however, they have not garnered significant clinical acceptance to date.

Summary
• Computer technology that automates test performance and reporting, controls data input and signal processing, and allows sophisticated ST-segment analysis is incorporated into all modern stress ECG systems.
• Complex data processing algorithms perform signal averaging and noise reduction so that the maximal amount of diagnostic information can be derived from the stress ECG.
• With properly obtained and processed signal-averaged data, digital measurements have been shown to be more accurate and more reproducible than simple visual assessments of the ST-segment response to stress.
• Various computer-derived ST-segment indexes in selected populations have been studied and proposed to enhance the diagnostic yield and limit the number of false-negative exercise ECG stress tests. However, these criteria have largely failed to achieve widespread clinical acceptance.
• Central to proper interpretation of computer-derived ECG data is good signal input with adequate skin preparation and reasoned clinical judgment to interpret test results in the context of the clinical situation.

References

Diamond, G.A., Staniloff, H.M., Forrester, J.S. et al. (1983). Computer-assisted diagnosis in the noninvasive evaluation of patients with suspected coronary artery disease. *J. Am. Coll. Cardiol.* 1 (2 Pt 1): 444–455.

Do, D., West, J.A., Morise, A. et al. (1997). A consensus approach to diagnosing coronary artery disease based on clinical and exercise test data. *Chest* 111: 1742–1749.

Firoozabadi, R., Gregg, R.E., and Babaeizadeh, S. (2016). Identification of exercise-induced ischemia using QRS slopes. *J. Electrocardiol.* 49: 55–59.

Hollenberg, M., Budge, W.R., Wisneski, J.A., and Gertz, E.W. (1980). Treadmill score quantifies electrocardiographic response to exercise and improves test accuracy and reproducibility. *Circulation* 61: 276–285.

Kligfield, P., Ameisen, O., and Okin, P.M. (1989). Heart rate adjustment of ST segment depression for improved detection of coronary artery disease. *Circulation* 79: 245–255.

Lehtinen, R., Sievänen, H., Viik, J. et al. (1996). Accurate detection of coronary artery disease by integrated analysis of the ST-segment depression/heart rate patterns during the exercise and recovery phases of the exercise electrocardiography test. *Am. J. Cardiol.* 78: 1002–1006.

McHenry, P.L., Phillips, J.F., and Knoebel, S.B. (1972). Correlation of computer-quantitated treadmill exercise electrocardiogram with arteriographic location of coronary artery disease. *Am. J. Cardiol.* 30: 747–752.

Okin, P.M., Anderson, K.M., Levy, D., and Kligfield, P. (1991). Heart rate adjustment of exercise-induced ST segment depression. Improved risk stratification in the Framingham Offspring Study. *Circulation* 83: 866–874.

Okin, P.M. and Kligfield, P. (1995). Heart rate adjustment of ST segment depression and performance the exercise electrocardiogram: a critical evaluation. *J. Am. Coll. Cardiol.* 25: 1726–1735.

Raxwal, V., Shetler, K., Morise, A. et al. (2001). Simple treadmill score to diagnose coronary disease. *Chest* 119: 1933–1940.

Sharir, T., Merzon, K., Kruchin, I. et al. (2012). Use of electrocardiographic depolarization abnormalities for detection of stress-induced ischemia as defined by myocardial perfusion imaging. *Am. J. Cardiol.* 109: 642–650.

Sheffield, L.T., Holt, J.H., Lester, F.M. et al. (1969). On-line analysis of the exercise electrocardiogram. *Circulation* 40: 935–944.

Simoons, M.L. and Hugenholtz, P.G. (1977). Estimation of the probability of exercise-induced ischemia by quantitative ECG analysis. *Circulation* 56 (4 Pt 1): 552–559.

21   Medicolegal Aspects of Stress ECG Testing

Dennis A. Tighe

Introduction

Stress testing is a non-invasive procedure which provides important diagnostic, functional, and prognostic assessment of patients with a variety of cardiovascular disorders. Though stress ECG testing is, in general, a safe procedure, certain procedural risks and complications of testing are recognized. To perform stress testing in a safe and efficient manner with a minimal risk of complications, certain procedures and guidelines must be followed. It is important that the stress laboratory be well designed and efficient in operation, that medical personnel be experienced and adequately trained, that appropriate screening for indications and contraindications of testing occur, that all laboratory protocols be closely followed, that necessary equipment be fully operational, and that appropriate personnel be immediately available should any emergency arise. This chapter briefly reviews these requirements as they relate to stress testing, as well potential medicolegal issues.

Pocket Guide to Stress Testing, Second Edition. Edited by Dennis A. Tighe and Bryon A. Gentile.
© 2020 John Wiley & Sons Ltd. Published 2020 by John Wiley & Sons Ltd.

The Stress Laboratory

- The area in which stress ECG testing is performed should be large enough to accommodate all necessary equipment and personnel.
- The laboratory area must have immediate access to full resuscitation equipment, including a defibrillator and emergency "crash-cart." The defibrillator should be inspected each day and the "crash-cart" should be inspected on a periodic basis per institutional standards. Documentation of this periodic inspection should be maintained.
- The laboratory should be equipped with a well-functioning cardiac monitoring system, allowing continuous print-out of rhythm strips and 12-lead ECGs. This system should conform to the specifications recommended by the American Heart Association.
- Written protocols governing all aspects of laboratory function should be established by the medical director of the stress ECG laboratory. All laboratory personnel should be completely familiar with these protocols and should follow them closely.

Medical Personnel

- A variety of medical personnel including physicians and non-physicians (technicians, clinical exercise physiologists, physician assistants, nurse practitioners, and registered nurses) may participate in the performance and/or supervision of a stress test.

Lab Personnel

- It is quite clear that stress testing should only be performed under the supervision of appropriately trained and experienced personnel with a fundamental knowledge of exercise physiology and ability to recognize important changes in rhythm and repolarization on the ECG. Appropriate certification from professional societies documenting clinical training and competencies in stress testing is mandatory. A minimum of training in basic life support (BLS) is required of all personnel working in our laboratory. Training in advanced cardiac life support (ACLS) and emergency cardiovascular care (ECC) is required of all licensed independent practitioners supervising stress testing in our laboratory.

Supervising Provider

- In general, current practice in most stress laboratories is that a physician does not directly supervise every stress test. It should be kept in mind, however, that the physician supervising the stress testing laboratory bears ultimate responsibility for all aspects of a stress test whether or not he/she directly performs the test. This includes proper test selection (see Chapters 3, 4, and 11), timely and accurate interpretation and reporting of testing data (see Chapter 14), and delivery of appropriate emergency care.
- In situations where high-risk patients (such as those post-recent myocardial infarction (MI), stabilized heart failure (HF), complex arrhythmia, unstable angina after medical stabilization, asymptomatic severe aortic stenosis, hypertrophic cardiomyopathy, significant pulmonary hypertension, or ion channelopathies) are referred for stress testing, it is imperative that these patients be identified and that a physician directly supervises the stress test.
- The physician supervising the stress testing laboratory should be immediately available should any potential difficulty, question regarding safety of test performance, appropriateness of test selection, or complication of testing arise.

Medical Director

- The medical director of the stress testing laboratory is responsible for ensuring the adequacy of the testing equipment, providing that the laboratory staff is properly trained and supervised, supplying clearly defined written protocols for safe and efficient laboratory operation and test performance, and developing a continuous quality assurance program for the laboratory. The medical director should insure that appropriate policies and procedures are followed and that regular emergency practice with documentation is conducted.

Test Preparation (see Chapters 2 and 3)

- A written request (order) for a stress test from the referring provider should accompany the patient.
- Prior to testing a brief history, physical examination, and inspection of a standard resting 12-lead ECG should be performed. These preparations are necessary to determine the appropriate form of stress testing and if contraindications to testing exist.

History and Physical Examination

- The history and physical examination are focused toward the cardiovascular system and the stated reason for test referral. In addition, the supervising provider should inquire about any serious non-cardiac condition[s] which may limit or prevent testing.
  - Historical and/or physical findings of an accelerating pattern of angina pectoris, recent MI, uncontrolled HF, serious arrhythmia, uncontrolled systemic hypertension, serious valvular heart disease, acute pulmonary embolism or infarction, acute deep venous thrombosis, suspected aortic dissection, infective endocarditis, myoperi-carditis, or any serious non-cardiac condition would be sufficient to cancel the stress test until further evaluation and therapy have occurred.

Medication History

- A careful history of both prescription and non-prescription medications should be obtained so that potential false positive or negative responses can be anticipated.

Resting ECG

- A standard, resting 12-lead ECG is required prior to testing and should be compared to a baseline tracing if available. In our experience cases of recent MI have been discovered, for which stress testing was contraindicated. In addition, if the Mason-Likar ("torso") 12-lead exercise configuration is used to obtain the resting ECG, we have noted that cases of inferior Q-wave MI can be missed as this arrangement shifts the frontal plane axis to the right, potentially increasing voltage in the inferior leads.

Explanation of the Test

- Following this brief, but important evaluation, the entire procedure of stress testing should be explained to the patient. In some cases, a brief demonstration of actual walking on a treadmill may be valuable.

Informed Consent

- Full and informed written consent should be obtained and placed in the medical record. For non-English-speaking patients, translation service should be provided; it is not sufficient to request that a family member or hospital employee fluent in the language of the patient be used to obtain this consent. The major risks of stress testing should be emphasized and explained to the patient in a manner that they can understand. The risk of death with stress testing ranges from 0.5 to 1.0/10 000 tests. MI may occur in 2–3/10 000 tests. The risk of serious complications may be higher among populations with higher prevalence of disease. Table 21.1 lists the various complications associated with stress testing. An example of an informed consent document for the non-treadmill stress ECG test is given in Table 21.2. (See Table 2.2 for an informed consent document for the treadmill stress test.)

Table 21.1 Complications of stress testing.

Cardiac complications
    Cardiac arrhythmias
        Tachyarrhythmias
            Atrial
            Atrioventricular junctional
            Ventricular
        Bradyarrhythmias
            Sinus
            Atrioventricular junctional
            Ventricular
            Atrioventricular block
            Asystole
    Angina pectoris
    Myocardial infarction
    Sudden death (ventricular tachycardia/fibrillation)
    Heart failure
    Hypertension
    Hypotension and shock
Noncardiac complications
    Musculoskeletal injury
    Vascular claudication
    Retinal separation

Phlebitis

Bronchospasm

Ill-defined and miscellaneous complications

Severe fatigue

Dizziness

General malaise

Fainting

Body ache

Flushing

Headache

Test Performance

- Proper written protocols for each type of stress test should exist in the laboratory and should be followed as closely as possible by the individual supervising the test.
- The proper exercise protocol or pharmacological stress test should be selected based upon patient characteristics by the supervising health-care professional (see Chapter 11).

Patient Monitoring

- During performance of the test and in recovery, blood pressure (BP), heart rate (HR) and rhythm, and ST-segment response to stress must be closely monitored. The test supervisor should be aware of patient symptoms. Awareness of these parameters is especially important during the early stages of exercise so that potential untoward effects can be prevented or minimized.

Table 21.2 Procedure consent form for non-treadmill stress ECG test.

---

1) I hereby authorize (Physician's Name) to perform upon (Patient's Name) the following medical procedure(s): (State specific name and nature of the procedure(s) to be performed).

2) I understand that the procedure(s) will be performed at (**Hospital Name**), by or under the supervision of (**Physician's Name**), who is authorized to utilize the services of other physicians and providers (e.g. **Cardiology Fellows, Nurse Practitioners, Physician Assistants, Exercise Physiologists, Nurses**).

3) I consent to the performance of procedure(s) different from those listed above, which my physician considers necessary or advisable in the course of the procedure(s).

4) I understand the nature and purpose of the procedure(s), possible alternative methods of diagnosis, the risks involved, the possibility of complications, and the consequences of the procedure(s). I acknowledge that no guarantee or assurance has been made to me as to the results that may be obtained.

5) I certify that I have read and fully understand the above consent statement. In addition, I have been afforded an opportunity to ask whatever questions I might have regarding the procedure(s) to be performed and they have been answered to my satisfaction.

_____   _____

Patient or Authorized Representative   Witness

(State Relationship to Patient)

_____   _____

Physician/Provider Obtaining Signature   Date/Time

- In our experience, careful notation of the patient's general appearance, breathing pattern, and facial expression by an experienced observer can detect patients who are nearing the limit of their exercise capacity. These observations can help to prevent adverse effects from further stress despite no significant ECG changes.
- Absolute indications for terminating a stress test (see Chapters 19) such as stress-induced hypotension, severe ECG changes, serious arrhythmia, chest discomfort, patient request, and technical difficulties should be closely followed.
- Other potential (relative) indications for terminating stress should be individualized by the test supervisor in to maximize diagnostic yield while maintaining patient safety.

Recovery Phase

- Close monitoring of the patient's ECG and vital signs should continue during recovery as abnormal responses may occur during this phase. The patient should be monitored for a minimum of six minutes after stress or until symptoms, vital signs, and ECG changes have reverted to near baseline. If symptoms, abnormal vital signs, or ECG changes persist beyond 15–20 minutes of recovery, we recommend hospital admission for the patient.
- A timely written interpretation of the stress test results should be available, ideally within 72 hours or less. A preliminary test reading, however, should be available immediately.
- The referring provider should be notified immediately per institutional standards of any complication or markedly abnormal response to stress.

Proper Emergency Equipment and Drugs

- All stress ECG laboratories should as a minimum have available the following emergency equipment:
  - Portable DC defibrillator
  - Oxygen and delivery devices (nasal cannula, mask)

- Suctioning apparatus
- "Crash cart" containing proper drugs, solutions, and equipment for ECC (Table 21.3)
- Needles, syringes, intravenous cannulas
- Bag-valve-mask type respirator (Ambu bag)
- Board for cardiac compression
- Equipment required for tracheal intubation (laryngoscope, endotracheal tubes)

Inspections

- This emergency equipment should be regularly inspected (the defibrillator should be turned on and discharged before each stress testing session) to ensure proper function. Emergency medications should be reviewed frequently so that none are past their listed expiration date. A record should be kept that documents these checks.

Staff

- All stress laboratory staff should be completely familiar with the location and operation of emergency equipment. A written protocol for staff response during emergency situations should exist, both for the stress laboratory and the institution where the laboratory is located.

Medico-legal Aspects as they Pertain to Stress ECG Testing

Despite adequate preparations, precautions, and compliance with the guidelines listed above for prudent and safe operation of a stress testing laboratory, complications can and will arise in conjunction with the performance of a

Table 21.3 Contents of code blue crash cart for stress ECG laboratory.

Emergency Medications	
Adenosine	6 mg/2 ml
Amiodarone	150 mg/3 ml
Aspirin	81 mg
Atropine sulfate	1 mg/10 ml syringe
Calcium chloride 10%	1 g/10 ml syringe
Dextrose 50%	25 g/50 ml syringe
Diazepam	10 mg/2 ml vial
Digoxin	0.5 mg/2 ml ampule
Diltiazem	20 mg vial
Diphenhydramine	50 mg/1 ml ampule
Dopamine	400 mg/250 ml (premixed)
Epinephrine 1:1000	1 ml ampule
Epinephrine 1:10 000	1 mg/1 ml syringe (1.5 in. needle)
Flumazenil	0.5 mg/ml
Furosemide	40 mg/4 ml vial (10 mg/ml)
Glucagon	1 mg vial
Isoproterenol 1:5000	1 mg/5 ml ampule
Lidocaine	100 mg/5 ml syringe

(*Continued*)

Table 21.3 (Continued)

Lidocaine 2%	30 ml vial (without epinephrine)
Lidocaine	2 g/250 ml (premixed)
Magnesium Sulfate	1 g/2 ml vial
Metoprolol	5 mg/5 ml
Naloxone	4 mg/10 ml vial (0.4 mg/ml)
Nitroglycerin	100 mg/250 ml (premixed)
Nitroglycerin	0.4 mg tablets
Norepinephrine	4 mg/4 ml
Phenytoin	100 mg/2 ml vial
Procainamide	1 g/10 ml vial (100 mg/ml)
Sodium bicarbonate 8.4%	50 meq/50 ml syringe
Solumedrol	125 mg vial
Succinylcholine	200 mg/10 ml vial
Vasopressin	20 units/ml; 1 ml vial
Normal Saline	30 cc vial
Bacteriostatic water	30 cc vial
Heparin flush	10 cc vial
Intravenous solutions	
Normal saline	1000 ml
Normal saline	250 ml

Lactated Ringer's	1000 ml
5% dextrose	250 ml
Emergency equipment	
Adhesive tape	Laryngoscope handle
Airways (oral and nasal)	Lubricant jelly
Alcohol wipes	Magill forceps
Alligator clamps	Medication labels
Ambu bag	Nasal cannula
Angiocaths (various sizes)	Nasopharyngeal airway
Batteries, sizes C and D	Needles and syringes (various sizes including cardiac needle)
Benzocaine spray	Needle box
Benzoine	Needle holder
Betadine swabs	Pacing box
Bite sticks	Pacing catheters
Bladder catheters	Protective clothing and goggles
Blades – curved (Macintosh size 3 and 4)	Salem sump tube
Blades – straight (Miller size 3 and 4)	Scalpel
Blood gas kits	Stopcocks
Bulbs (flashlight and laryngoscope)	Stylettes
CO_2 colorimetric indicator	Suction catheters

(Continued)

Table 21.3 (Continued)

CVP kit including introducer sheathes	Suction device with tubing
Defibrillator/monitor and pads	Suture material
ECG leads and electrodes	Syringes
Endotracheal tubes (various sizes)	Tongue depressors
External pacemaker and pads	Tourniquets
Flashlight	Tracheotomy tray
Gauze pads	Tubing for IV solutions
Gloves (sterile and nonsterile)	Vacutainer device
IV pole	Venous cut-down tray
Laboratory tubes for blood	Worksheet

stress ECG test. Should a complication arise, compliance with proper procedures, a full and informed consent, and good documentation will minimize but not completely eradicate the risk of legal action against healthcare professionals or the stress testing laboratory.

Basis of Legal Action

- A legal action against a healthcare professional or a stress testing laboratory can involve charges of battery and/or negligence.
- *Battery* may be defined simply as the "unconsented touching" of a patient. Interestingly, battery is often excluded in malpractice insurance policies and often is not part of a medical malpractice suit.

- *Negligence* is defined as care that falls below an expected, reasonable standard which exists in the community. To establish negligence four conditions must be met:
  1) A pre-existing duty (responsibility to provide care) was present.
  2) A breach of duty (action contrary to the recognized standard of medical practice) occurred.
  3) Damages (injury) must exist. These damages may be physical, emotional, and/or financial.
  4) A proximate cause (causal link) must exist between the breach of duty and damages that resulted.
- All four conditions must be present to establish negligence; however, damages without a clear breach of duty does not qualify as negligence.

Informed Consent and Minimization of Risk

The stress ECG test is an elective diagnostic procedure. In dealing with elective diagnostic procedures the healthcare professional has two basic responsibilities:

1) The patient must be made aware of foreseeable risks of that procedure, and with such knowledge he/she consents to it.
2) The procedure should be carefully performed and all steps to minimize risk to the patient should be taken.

Informed Consent

- The first responsibility is *informed consent*, legally defined as "a reasonable disclosure to the patient of the nature of his/her disease, of the treatment, and of the probable consequences of the treatment."
- A stress ECG test should not be performed without first explaining the nature of the procedure and its potential risks, as discussed above, to the patient and then obtaining an informed consent document signed by the patient and witnessed by the supervising healthcare professional.

Minimize Risk

- The second responsibility of the supervising healthcare professional is to select the technique most likely to provide the required information at the lowest possible risk to the patient.
- A stress ECG test should be supervised by medical personnel highly trained in test administration and skilled in recognition and treatment of complications and emergency situations. The laboratory and its equipment should be functioning properly. Clearly defined procedures and policies should be rigorously followed.

Non-physician Medical Personnel

- The role of medical personnel other than the supervising physician are less well defined from a medico-legal standpoint. It is in general agreement that only a physician may diagnose, treat, assess the progress of disease, or perform complex procedures on the human body.
- Most contemporary stress testing laboratories assign the duty of stress test administration and immediate aftercare (excepting the highest-risk patients) to non-physician medical personnel. The physician is completely responsible for selecting trained and competent assistants and maintaining quality and safety.
  - These non-physician personnel must be fully familiar with the procedure, including its indications and contraindications. In addition, they are obligated to act only within the scope of their practice, as defined by professional certifying bodies.
  - Depending upon the circumstances, the physician may be legally responsible for malpractice along with these non-physicians for breach of duty or negligence on their part.
  - At the present time, a non-physician, no matter how well trained, may not and should not be the sole administrator of a stress ECG test; physician oversight at an appropriate level is required.
  - From the medico-legal point of view, the physician responsible for test supervision and/or the physician-in-charge of the stress testing laboratory are completely responsible for the entire procedure, including final test interpretation.

Summary

- Fully trained and competent laboratory personnel, properly functioning equipment, and readily available emergency cardiac care provisions are mandatory to minimize the risk of complications and ensure safe performance of stress ECG testing.
- Each patient must be assessed individually for appropriate test indications, potential contraindications, and proper test selection to minimize risk.
- Informed consent is a mandatory process before the performance of a stress ECG test.
- The stress testing laboratory should be supervised by a competent, well-trained, and experienced physician who is immediately available when needed and required.
- Strict adherence to laboratory policies and procedures established by the medial director and institution where the test is conducted will minimize the risk of provider/laboratory liability in threatened legal action.
- The ultimate responsibility for all aspects of the stress ECG test belongs to the supervising physician, whether or not he/she directly administers the test.

References

Myerburg, R.J., Chaitman, B.R., Ewy, G.A., and Lauer, M.S. (2008). Task force 2: training in electrocardiography, ambulatory electrocardiography, and exercise testing. *J. Am. Coll. Cardiol.* 51: 348–354.

Myers, J., Arena, R., Franklin, B. et al., on behalf of the American Heart Association Committee on Exercise, Cardiac Rehabilitation, and Prevention of the Council on Clinical Cardiology, the Council on Nutrition, Physical Activity, and Metabolism, and the Council on Cardiovascular Nursing (2009). Recommendations for clinical exercise laboratories: a scientific statement from the American Heart Association. *Circulation* 119: 3144–3161.

Myers, J., Forman, D.E., Balady, G.J. et al., American Heart Association Subcommittee on Exercise, Cardiac Rehabilitation, and Prevention of the Council on Clinical Cardiology, Council on Lifestyle and Cardiometabolic Health, Council on Epidemiology and Prevention, and Council on Cardiovascular and Stroke Nursing (2014). Supervision of exercise testing by nonphysicians: a scientific statement from the American Heart Association. *Circulation* 130: 1014–1027.

Rodgers, G.P., Ayanian, J.Z., Balady, G. et al. (2000). American College of Cardiology/American Heart Association clinical competence statement on stress testing: a report of the American College of Cardiology/American Heart Association/American College of Physicians-American Society of Internal Medicine Task Force on Clinical Competence. *Circulation* 102: 1726–1738.

22 Educational Guide for Patients and Families

Dennis A. Tighe

Introduction

The purpose of this chapter is to provide a simple and concise guide to the various types of stress tests offered in the stress ECG testing laboratory that will help patients and their families in understanding these tests. We describe each test in sufficient detail so that patients and their families can comprehend what is expected before, during, and after the stress test. We have found that a similar such guide, available in written and online forms, used in our laboratory has answered many patient and family questions and has led to better understanding of what a stress test entails. Patients and family are asked in advance to read the sections which correspond to the test requested by their referring physician. Patients and their families are encouraged to contact the stress laboratory if unanswered questions remain. For more specific or complex questions that involve patient-related issues (example: which medication[s] should be taken the day of testing), the patient and/or family is requested to speak to the referring provider.

Pocket Guide to Stress Testing, Second Edition. Edited by Dennis A. Tighe and Bryon A. Gentile.

Exercise ECG (Treadmill) Stress Test

Background on the Test

- If your provider feels that you can walk briskly enough to achieve an adequate heart rate (HR) and level of exercise, you will be asked to undergo a treadmill exercise electrocardiographic (ECG) test.
- The purpose of this test is to evaluate the function of your heart, the adequacy of your heart medications, and/or to prescribe an activity program for you.
- The treadmill exercise ECG test involves a team of certified healthcare professionals lead by a physician (cardiologist) that also includes nurses, physician assistants, exercise physiologists, and technicians. Each team member has special training in this area.

Your Preparation for the Test

- Please consult with your referring provider as to which medication(s) you should or should not take prior to your test.
- You should plan to be at the hospital for one to two hours. Do not eat or drink anything for at least three hours prior to your test, except for medications (if any) that you regularly take with small sips of water.
- On the day of your test, wear comfortable walking shoes (preferably sneakers), loose-fitting pants or shorts, and a blouse or shirt with buttons that opens in the front.
- Please bring your medications or a complete list of all your medications (drug name, dose, and frequency) with you to avoid delay.

When You Arrive for the Test

- When you arrive at the stress testing laboratory a technician will verify that an order exists for the test and its indication. The technician will ask you about your current medications.
- Prior to the test, ECG electrodes will be placed on your chest. For men, this may require removal of chest hair. A brief medical history and examination will then be performed by the test supervisor.

Taking the Test

- During this test we will ask you to walk on a motor-driven treadmill. While a "target HR," based on your age, is a goal of testing, we ask that you exercise as much as you can.
- The speed and incline of the treadmill will gradually increase every three (3) minutes.
- Your HR, blood pressure (BP), and ECG will be closely monitored throughout the test by our team.
- It is important that you concentrate during the test and attempt to exercise as long as possible. Walking for as long as possible gives your referring provider the most information about the function of your heart. The test supervisor may periodically ask you about how you are feeling during the exercise bout. The test will be stopped if you have any significant symptoms, the test supervisor believes that enough information has been obtained, or you request the test to stop.
- After exercise, we will closely monitor your HR, BP, and ECG for a few minutes while you recover.

After the Test Is Completed

- Following completion of the test, we will remove the electrodes.
- Provided no further testing is required, you are free to leave the testing laboratory.
- Your referring provider will receive a complete report of your test.

Exercise-Myocardial Perfusion Imaging ("Nuclear") Scan

Background on the Test

- When the treadmill exercise ECG test alone is not sufficient to diagnose your heart condition or when additional information is needed, your referring provider may request a myocardial perfusion imaging ("nuclear") scan in addition to your exercise ECG stress test. This test helps to determine how much blood is received by your heart during exercise and at rest.

Your Preparations for the Test

- Please refer to the information above regarding the exercise ECG (treadmill) stress test for preparations and details of that test.
- Do not eat or drink anything the morning of your test(s). Regularly scheduled medications can be taken with small sips of water. Please consult with your referring provider about which medication(s) should or should not be taken prior to the test.
- Since nuclear scanning requires additional preparations and equipment, please allow four to five hours for testing the day of the exercise test. In most cases, exercise and rest scanning will be completed on the same day. Please do not eat anything between scans unless directed by a member of our team.

Taking the Test

- The myocardial perfusion imaging test involves placement of a small catheter in a vein and injection of a radioactive tracer substance just before the end of exercise. In most cases, a separate injection at rest is required. The radioactive tracer has no significant side effects.

- Just after exercise you will be asked to lie under a special camera for thirty (30) minutes to obtain exercise scan images.
- Depending upon which radiotracer substance you receive and/or protocol followed, rest images may be scheduled to be obtained before exercise, within three to four hours after completion of exercise or arranged for the following morning.
- If a rest scan is required the following day, please do not eat anything the morning of the test. When you arrive, an intravenous (IV) catheter will be started, the tracer agent will be injected, and 45–60 minutes later scanning will be performed. Plan to be at the hospital for about two (2) hours.

After the Test Is Completed

- Following completion of the test, we will remove the electrodes and the IV catheter.
- Provided no further testing is required, you are free to leave the testing laboratory.
- Your referring provider will receive a complete report of your test results.

Vasodilator (Adenosine, Dipyridamole, or Regadenoson) Cardiac Perfusion Test

Background on the Test

- A vasodilator perfusion stress test is recommended by your provider when it is anticipated that you cannot perform a treadmill exercise ECG stress test to an adequate level. This test does not involve physical exercise, such as walking or pedaling a bicycle, but requires the infusion of chemical agent (the "vasodilator") over a short time period in order to increase blood flow to the heart. A myocardial perfusion imaging ("nuclear") scan (see "Exercise-Myocardial Perfusion Imaging ('Nuclear') Scan" above) is required with this test.

- The vasodilator perfusion test involves a team of physicians (cardiologists), nurses, and technicians. Each team member has special training in this area.

Your Preparations for the Test

- Since nuclear scanning requires additional preparations and equipment, please allow four to five hours for testing on the day of the perfusion stress test. In most cases, stress and rest scanning will be completed in one day. Please do not eat anything between scans unless directed by a member of our team.
- Do not eat or drink anything for at least three hours before your test(s). Please consult with your referring provider about which medication(s) should or should not be taken prior to the test. Regularly scheduled medications can be taken with small sips of water. Please do not take Persantine (dipyridamole), Aggrenox, Theophylline (Slo-bid, Slophylline, etc.), or Trental (pentoxifylline) for 24–48 hours prior to the test as these medications may interfere with the actions of the agent used for the stress portion of the test.
- In addition, a variety of other prescription medications (Fiorinal, Fioricet, Cafergot) and over-the-counter (non-prescription) medications, including but not limited to Anacin, Excedrin, Dexatrim, and Dristan, contain caffeine, which interferes with the actions of the agent used for the stress portion of the test. It is advised that you check with your referring provider about which medications should be discontinued prior to testing.
- You should also refrain from consuming beverages, foods, and other products containing caffeine, including coffee, teas, colas, chocolate, diet supplements, energy drinks, and products containing guarana, for a minimum of 12–24 hours prior to testing.
- Infusion of a vasodilator agent is not advised for patients with a history of asthma, wheezing, or those using inhalers to help their breathing. Please inform the test supervisor of any of these conditions prior to your test.
- Please bring your medications or a complete list of all your medications (drug name, dose, and frequency) with you to avoid delay.

When You Arrive for the Test

- When you arrive at the stress testing laboratory a technician will verify the order for your stress test and ask about your current medications.
- Prior to the test, ECG electrodes will be placed on your chest. For men, this may require removal of chest hair. A brief medical history and examination will then be performed by the test supervisor.

Taking the Test

- This test requires that one or two intravenous (IV) lines be inserted for infusion/injection of the vasodilator agent and injection of the myocardial perfusion tracer.
- During this test you will lie on a table while the vasodilator agent is administered. The myocardial perfusion agent will be injected during the test by a technician. Your HR, BP, and ECG will be closely monitored throughout the test by our team. This portion of the test lasts approximately fifteen (15) minutes.
- The test supervisor will ask you about side effects from the medication; please inform him/her if you experience chest discomfort, shortness of breath, nausea or any other sensation abnormal for you.

After the Test

- Following completion of the test, we will remove the ECG electrodes and the IV catheter.
- Myocardial perfusion ("nuclear") scanning will then start and you will lie under a special camera for approximately 20–30 minutes.
- Depending upon which radiotracer substance you receive, rest images may be scheduled to be obtained before administration of the stress agent, within three to four hours after completion of the first scan or arranged for the

following morning. In most cases, stress and rest scanning will be completed on the same day. Please do not eat anything between scans unless directed by a member of our team.

- If a rest scan is required the following day, please do not eat anything the morning of the test. When you arrive, an intravenous (IV) catheter will be started, the myocardial perfusion imaging ("nuclear") agent will be injected, and 45–60 minutes later scanning will be performed. Plan to be at the hospital for about two (2) hours.
- Your doctor will receive a complete report of your test results.

Dobutamine Myocardial Perfusion Imaging ("Nuclear") Stress Test

Background on the Test

- A dobutamine cardiac perfusion imaging stress test is recommended when it is anticipated that you cannot perform a treadmill exercise ECG stress test to an adequate level. This test does not involve physical exercise such as walking or pedaling a bicycle, but requires the infusion of a progressively increasing dose of dobutamine over a short time period, which will chemically simulate exercise. A myocardial perfusion imaging ("nuclear") scan (please see above) is required with this test.
- The dobutamine perfusion stress test is conducted a team of physicians (cardiologists), nurses, and technicians. Each team member has special training in this area.

Your Preparations for the Test

- Do not eat or drink anything for at least three hours prior to your test(s). Regularly scheduled medications can be taken with small sips of water. Please consult with your referring provider about which medication(s) should or should not be taken prior to the test.

- Since nuclear scanning requires additional preparations and equipment, please allow four to five hours for testing the day of the dobutamine perfusion stress test. In most cases, stress and rest scanning will be completed in one day. Please do not eat anything between scans unless directed by a member of our team.
- Please bring your medications or a complete list of all your medications (drug name, dose, and frequency) with you to avoid delay.

When You Arrive for the Test

- When you arrive at the stress testing laboratory a technician will verify the order and indication for the test and ask you about your current medications.
- Prior to the test, ECG electrodes will be placed on your chest. For men, this may require removal of chest hair. A brief medical history and examination will then be performed by the test supervisor.

Taking the Test

- The test requires that one intravenous (IV) line be inserted for infusion of dobutamine and injection of the myocardial perfusion imaging ("nuclear") agent.
- During this test you will lie on a table while dobutamine is infused. The myocardial perfusion agent will be injected during the test by a technician. Your HR, BP, and ECG will be closely monitored throughout the test by our team. This portion of the test will last approximately thirty (30) minutes.
- The test supervisor will ask you periodically about side effects from the medication; please do not hesitate to inform him/her if you experience chest discomfort, heart pounding, shortness of breath, nausea, flushing, headache, or feel anxious.

- Following completion of the dobutamine infusion, we will continue to monitor your HR, BP, and ECG. When your vital signs and ECG have returned to normal, we will remove the electrodes. Myocardial perfusion ("nuclear") scanning will then start, during which you will lie under a special camera for approximately 20–30 minutes.
- Depending upon which radiotracer substance you receive, rest images may be scheduled to be obtained prior to infusion of dobutamine, within three to four hours after completion of the first scan or arranged for the following morning.
- If a rest scan is required the following day, please do not eat anything the morning of the test. When you arrive, an intravenous (IV) catheter will be started, the myocardial perfusion agent will be injected, and the scan will be performed 45–60 minutes later. Plan to be at the hospital for about two (2) hours.
- Your doctor will receive a complete report of your test results.

Exercise Treadmill Test or Dobutamine Test with Echocardiography ("Stress Echocardiography")

Background on the Test

- Echocardiography (ultrasound or sound wave test) is an alternative to myocardial perfusion ("nuclear") imaging to evaluate heart function during stress. There are no known side effects from the type of ultrasound we use.
- The preparations for either an exercise ECG treadmill test or dobutamine infusion test are the same as for the other types of tests. See the other sections for test preparations.

Taking the Test

- The test procedure is slightly different when echocardiography is used. Sound wave images are first obtained when you are resting. The technician will apply gel (may be cool) to the sound wave transducer and then place this transducer on your chest in order to visualize the heart. A small amount of pressure may be felt when the transducer is in contact with your chest. The technician will record appropriate images in four different views with supervision from the test supervisor.

- Once these views of the heart have been obtained, the stress test will be performed. Please refer to the appropriate section above for details of the test procedure.

Exercise Treadmill Stress Echocardiography

Preparations for the Test

- You should plan to be at the hospital for one to two hours.
- Do not eat or drink anything for at least three hours prior to your test, except for medications (if any) that you regularly take with small sips of water.
- Please consult with your referring provider as to which of your medication(s) you should continue to take prior to your test.
- On the day of your test, wear comfortable walking shoes (preferably sneakers), loose-fitting pants or shorts, and a blouse or shirt with buttons that opens in the front.

Taking the Test

- For the exercise treadmill test, you will be asked to exercise for as long as possible. Your HR, BP, and ECG will be closely monitored throughout the test by our team.
- After the exercise bout ("stress"), you will be directed by members of our team to return to the bed as quickly as possible so that echocardiography can be repeated in the same views as before exercise.
- After exercise and the stress imaging is completed, we will closely monitor your vital signs and ECG for a few minutes while you recover.

After the Test

- Following completion of the test, we will remove the ECG electrodes.
- Provided no further testing is required, you are free to leave the testing laboratory.
- Your doctor will receive a complete report of your test.

Dobutamine Stress Echocardiography

Preparations for the Test

- You should plan to be at the hospital for about two hours.
- Do not eat or drink anything for at least three hours prior to your test, except for medications (if any) that you regularly take with small sips of water.
- Please consult with your referring provider as to which of your medication(s) you should continue to take prior to your test.
- On the day of your test, please wear loose-fitting clothing, preferably a blouse or shirt with buttons that opens in the front.

Taking the Test

- Prior to infusion of the dobutamine the echocardiography technician will obtain sound wave images of your heart ("resting images").
- During dobutamine stress echocardiography, dobutamine will be infused as described in the section "Dobutamine Myocardial Perfusion Imaging ('Nuclear') Stress Test." Your HR, BP, and ECG will be closely monitored throughout the test by our team.

- During the dobutamine infusion and after its completion, the technician will periodically obtain ultrasound images of your heart and record them.
- After the infusion is done, we will closely monitor your vital signs and ECG for a few minutes while you recover.

After the Test

- Following completion of the test, we will remove the electrodes and the IV catheter.
- Provided no further testing is required, you are free to leave the testing laboratory.
- Your referring provider will receive a complete report of your test.

Important for All Tests

- If any of the following symptoms are present, please bring them to the attention of your provider before the test day. Please let our staff know if you are experiencing any of these symptoms on the day of your test.
- For all types of stress tests, please let your provider and our staff know if you are experiencing:
  - Chest, arm, jaw, or back pain/pressure/discomfort/heaviness at rest.
  - An increase in the frequency or severity of your chest symptoms.
  - Increasing shortness of breath.
  - Episodes of passing out.
  - Fever, increasing cough, or other signs of infection.
- Specifically for vasodilator (non-exercise) stress studies, please let us know if:
  - You have a history of asthma, emphysema, wheezing, inhaler use, or seizures.

Delays

- In the stress laboratory, as in most other specialty areas, unexpected emergency situations may occur which are beyond our control. If we know far enough in advance, we will make every effort to contact you to reschedule your appointment. On occasion there may also be an unavoidable delay in waiting time, but we will do our best to keep this to a minimum. We would like to thank you in advance for your patience and your cooperation. Please contact us at the stress laboratory if you have any questions.

Index

Pocket Guide to Stress Testing, Second Edition. Edited by Dennis A. Tighe and Bryon A. Gentile.
© 2020 John Wiley & Sons Ltd. Published 2020 by John Wiley & Sons Ltd.